New Life Hiking Spa®'s
40 years of
Authentic
Wellness

A Counter-Intuitive Personal Approach
to Letting Go of Dieting

Jimmy LeSage, M.S.

BALBOA.
PRESS
A DIVISION OF HAY HOUSE

Balboa Press books may be ordered through booksellers or by contacting:

Balboa Press
A Division of Hay House
1663 Liberty Drive
Bloomington, IN 47403
www.balboapress.com
1 (877) 407-4847

Because of the dynamic nature of the Internet, any web addresses or links contained in this book may have changed since publication and may no longer be valid. The views expressed in this work are solely those of the author and do not necessarily reflect the views of the publisher, and the publisher hereby disclaims any responsibility for them.

The author of this book does not dispense medical advice or prescribe the use of any technique as a form of treatment for physical, emotional, or medical problems without the advice of a physician, either directly or indirectly. The intent of the author is only to offer information of a general nature to help you in your quest for emotional and spiritual well-being. In the event you use any of the information in this book for yourself, which is your constitutional right, the author and the publisher assume no responsibility for your actions.

Any people depicted in stock imagery provided by Thinkstock are models, and such images are being used for illustrative purposes only.
Certain stock imagery © Thinkstock.

Print information available on the last page.

ISBN: 978-1-5043-9112-2 (sc)
ISBN: 978-1-5043-9113-9 (e)

Library of Congress Control Number: 2017916941

Balboa Press rev. date: 11/01/2017

CONTENTS

What Is New Life? ix

Foreword xi

Acknowledgments xiii

Introduction xv

Food and Eating Since the Mid-Twentieth Century xv

What This Is about and Who It's For xvi

Chapter 1: The Fundamentals 1

My Journey Begins 1

Who Was Nathan Pritikin? 4

A Historical Perspective on Our Relationship with Food 5

Let's Begin This Reeducation 6

The Food-Industrial Complex, Big Pharma, and Institutional Dieting .. 7

You Are the Focus 8

Chapter 2: The Education 10

I Will Be Your Guide 10

What Real Food Is 12

The Grocery Store 15

The Health Food Store 30

The Convenience Stores 31

The Institutional Pharmacy 32

Organic and Genetically Modified Organism (GMO) 33

Additives in Food 34

Vitamins and Dietary Supplements 34

Balanced Fitness 35

Chapter 3: The Sociology 39

How Much to Eat 41

Calories 42

The Rice Maker 44

Decisions at Restaurants 44

The "Only One Cookie" Situation 63

Chapter 4: The Psychology 66

Abundance Out of Control 66

Emotional Eating 67

A Deeper Understanding 68

Self-Discipline and Personal Responsibility 69

Weight and Other Measures 70

Chapter 5: The Practicalities 72

Jekyll and Hyde and the Pig-Out 72

Liquid Sugar Problem 74

Teas, Coffee, Carrot Juice, Juicing 76

Examples of how to read labels 77

Allergies, Fads, and Different Diets 82

Kitchen Suggestions 83

Ceramic Knife 85

Pots, Pans, and Other Kitchen Items 85

Recipe Conversions 86

Recipes—Jimmy's Favorites 97

Oatmeal Pancakes 100

Nuts: The Healthy Alternative to Health Bars 101

Studies and Claims 103

Our Children 105

Takeaways 105

A Recipe to Implement Authentic Wellness 109

Biography **111**

Childhood 111

Growing up in Florida to Working in Vermont Kitchens 112

Let the Off-Season Traveling Begin 115

Early New Life 118

Leaving Herbie's Kitchen 121

If I Can Make It There 121

I Can Make It Anywhere 123

Suitcase in Paradise 126

Talking the Talk 126

And Walking the Walk 127
Crossing the Divide...131
What More? 132
About the Author 133

WHAT IS NEW LIFE?

I, Jimmy LeSage, got the idea for the New Life Hiking Spa in 1977, and the organization will celebrate its fortieth anniversary in 2018. For readers of this book who don't know about the New Life Hiking Spa, it is important for you to have an overview. Opening in 1978, the New Life Hiking Spa, which is in the Green Mountains of Vermont, was one of the first destination spa wellness programs in the country. It is where people from all walks of life come to renew body and mind, eat healthy food, breathe the fresh, clean air of the mountains, and find physical and mental renewal in a wellness immersion and supportive atmosphere. Hikes, stretching, fitness classes, spa treatments, and three clean meals a day make up the basis of getting one's authentic wellness back on track. See the New Life Hiking Spa website for further details.

FOREWORD

Jimmy LeSage is a man on a continuing mission for forty years now. His mission is exceedingly difficult because it involves food, the most fundamental aspect of your health and survival. Jimmy's mission calls on you to examine your relationship with food. He wants to equip you to transform twentieth-century food understanding into one fitting for you in the twenty-first century.

Jimmy emphasizes the need for you to be the originator, the author of the transformation. Because your relationship with food is so vital to your health and at the same time so very personal, the *well-being* being sought is *authentic* solely to you.

Jimmy urges you to abandon many pillars of the food and eating culture established since the mid-twentieth century. In reforming your food relationship into its twenty-first-century version, you will learn of the insignificance, even harmfulness of concepts, methods, and assumptions associated with the food and eating culture since the midpoint of the twentieth century.

His approach offers you a path to your own well-being that frees you from diets, prescriptive regimes, food content, the mathematics of calories, or portion management, weight, and other data measures. Jimmy has told me that he yearns, even dreams that this book will end your focus on the previously mentioned concerns and the questions that derive from them. Instead, unshackled from irrelevancies remaining from your twentieth-century food relationship, you will be free to work toward your genuine well-being. Your twenty-first-century relationship with food will take form as you pursue your *authentic wellness*. On this path you will recognize yourself as the water-based being that you are, and you will acquire the understanding and the practical means to restore and preserve the purity of the water, which is the essence of your being.

My opportunity to participate as Jimmy's collaborator in this effort is the result of good fortune. I was in the right place when Jimmy felt driven to "get it all out." In effect, this was the point at which he chose to channel his deep-seated frustration with irrelevant questions into articulation of *authentic wellness.* Braced by the trust and respect forged during our relationship, he and I have explored complexities in your relationship with food and the changes that will improve and transform your well-being. Our hope is to convey these complexities clearly to create understanding in an approach that motivates you toward *authentic wellness.*

—Leonard Klepner

ACKNOWLEDGMENTS

New Life is my ongoing practice in the art and science of eating well and staying active. I have been doing New Life for forty years. During that period I have had hundreds of employees. All have contributed to New Life. They have demonstrated their commitment to New Life guests. As enlightened and skilled practitioners, they continue to advance New Life's wellness achievements. These employees have enhanced my understanding of the fitness and health practices in which they specialize. This is my sincere thanks to them all.

One of the advantages of a business operated in Vermont's off-season is that I have been able to provide quality employment to quality people. I have been blessed with great staff members from many different walks of life who have worked most closely with our guests over the years. I am proud of all that we have accomplished and will continue to accomplish at New Life for and with our guests. The guests who return repeatedly to share their experience with us are also very meaningful to me. The guests, too, deserve my utmost appreciation for joining their personal wellness journey to all involved with New Life.

I also want to deeply thank the love of my life, my wonderful and dedicated wife, Kathleen LeSage. With her on my team, New Life reached unimaginable new levels. Without her, our journey would not have brought us to the people and places so vital to New Life's success. Finally, I wish that I could speak adequately of the measure of richness and joy that Kathleen and our children, James and LeAnne, impart continuingly to our journey.

Finally, I share actualization of this book with my collaborators, Leonard Klepner and Cameron Sardelli. Each contributed respectively from our contrasting and complementary professional competencies to this effort. Leonard's immersion in the project began with ongoing discussion about my journey and my considered views about food, eating, fitness, and wellness. After the 2015 season inside New Life business operations as my assistant, Leonard was sufficiently socialized into life at New Life for us to initiate the project in earnest during New Life's 2016 season. Leonard has applied organizational judgment and narrative skills acquired over thirty years of professional engagement in the public administration of federal food and nutrition programs to transpose my thought and collected writings about achieving well-being into the concepts and presentation articulated by this book.

Cameron is a local Vermonter with his MBA. His commitment to personal fitness, outdoor activities and an authentic lifestyle is what brought us together on this project. He has spent his past five summers with New Life, and he has even admitted that he has learned new things about health and wellness each of those years. This book was an out-of-the-norm project for him. He says it really made him appreciate the New Life philosophy and opened his eyes to years of wellness wisdom that he can use throughout his life. Beyond the value of his perspective within the projects generational divide, he has enhanced the book with aesthetic, visual, and design sensibility. He constantly acted as a reminder to keep this project focused on the reader and how we can best share this fundamental, counterintuitive, and life-improving information. Cameron's research and input was the basis for several sections in this book.

INTRODUCTION

Food and Eating Since the Mid-Twentieth Century

This book is about the food we eat and the transformation that has unfolded with the baby boomer generation, of which I, Jimmy LeSage, born in 1950, have been a part. Since my birth, I have witnessed a period of unprecedented change in human history throughout every aspect of our lives—technology, society, environment, food, among many others. This book is about that change related to food. It presents a multidimensional strategy to navigate the food-related behaviors imposed on you individually and on our society.

Look around you—first at you own girth and then at the people present in all your life situations. There's no doubt that you are aware of the prevalence of degenerative diseases, such as diabetes, high blood pressure, heart attack, and stroke. I believe that a significant reason for this is the kind and amount of food (and nonfood) we consume. Unfortunately, the situation is getting worse rather than better. I recently read that since 1980, the number of obese Americans has doubled.

As with sleep, much of life is time we spend dealing with our food— not just eating it but getting it. Human existence may be understood as the effort required of us as food gatherers and hunters, as food cultivators, and most recently and only since the mid-twentieth century, as food processors and consumers of food that is not actually food. Like much else that has unfolded across recent history from the mid-twentieth century forward, our changed relationship with food has happened at an unprecedented rapid pace.

Our changed relationship with our food has included an onslaught of sugar, fat, salt, and unrecognizable and unpronounceable chemical, preservative, and taste-inducing ingredients. These substances have polluted the predominantly water-based purity of the creatures that we are. However, as evidenced by the increase in degenerative disease and the commonality of food-related allergies and sensitivities, our coping strategies have been ineffective at best and arguably even detrimental. Dieting, calorie consciousness, and countless other regimens and structural disciplines have not worked.

These remedies have not and cannot address our relationship with food comprehensively because that relationship, as indicated already, is multidimensional—that is, complex and the outcome of many influences. Our food relationship is also subjective—that is, very personal and individual, a behavior set determined by and comprising our lifestyles. The central focus of this book is to offer a unique understanding of your relationship with food and a path on which your acquired understanding will equip you to encounter and navigate twenty-first-century food issues. This path is the route toward and the experience of *authentic wellness*.

Who am I to address this situation and help you on a new path related to the most universal act that we all do, namely eat? To answer this question, I must ask you to allow me to present an overview of my life journey as it relates to food and general wellness. For more detail, read the extended biography at the end of this book. This will help you have a deeper understand how my journey evolved into the new perspective I am proposing.

What This Is about and Who It's For

This book presents the pursuit of the *authentic wellness* made possible with food and fitness through the perspectives of education, sociology, and psychology of eating. Mastering these aspects affords you the ability to individualize your pursuit of *authentic wellness*, giving you a new viewpoint of the tools to succeed. The understanding that the book conveys is applicable to you regardless of your wealth, age, or other distinction.

The multidimensional nature of the book's education, sociology, and psychology sections are made clear in the book's final section, "The Practicalities." There you will find pragmatic suggestions to consider for your lifestyle demands. Most importantly, the final section's topics and discussion will equip you to confront and navigate your lifestyle with self-tolerance.

More to the point, the book's principles seek to dispel food- and fitness-related thought, behaviors, and practices that have relentlessly ravaged our quality of life. The relationship we have with our food and fitness has dramatically changed in the United States since the mid-twentieth century, and it has proceeded to move globally as well. *Authentic wellness* is your route to restoring the purity of the water basis that all of us require preserving our essence as human beings.

CHAPTER 1

The Fundamentals

My Journey Begins

To embark on your own journey to *authentic wellness*, it will be helpful for you to understand the milestones I found on my own path.

The founding and ongoing changes that became New Life and the New Life Food Plan are two significant milestones to discover. When I started New Life, there were limited activities. The principle and virtually sole objective was weight loss. For the first few years, there wasn't even hiking.

In the mid-1980s, I started hearing guests talk about wanting to reduce stress and create a healthy lifestyle, but their continued impression was that weight loss was the way to do this. Late in the 1980s, I introduced an increased emphasis on health and the mind-body connection. These changes in emphasis were based mostly on my own cumulative knowledge, professional experiences, and observations of New Life guests' experiences. Weight loss was still the underlying reason guests came to New Life, but my interaction with guests made me sense that their faith in the value of dieting and weight loss was waning.

Indeed, the early 1990s broadened the focus of health beyond weight loss to lifestyle change. By the turn of the century, I was finally hearing guests say, "Diets don't work." And through their New Life experience, they wanted to acquire a deeper understanding of what a healthy lifestyle could be and to transfer the practices presented at New Life to their lifestyles to approximate their New Life experience. They were letting go of what I call "institutional dieting." As discussed throughout this book, my reference to "institutional dieting" encompasses any of the endless, usually commercial versions of structured, frequently programmatic responses to changing your relationship with food. Institutional dieting regimes range from mere fads to intricately prescribed behaviors and foods.

Although in my view the transition away from institutional dieting is becoming a major step toward a progressive and effective path to health, only in the last few years has the concept embodied by the term *wellness* become a true guest objective. The inspiration burning in the heart of New Life had always been about wellness. In contrast to weight loss, New Life preferred the pursuit of wellness more comprehensively through subjective lifestyle adaptation as it relates to food and other wellness considerations.

Evidence of the consistency and ongoing pertinence of New Life's food philosophy is the persistence of New Life's food ratio. When I started New Life, Black River Produce opened in the same year. The business included two guys and a station wagon. At the time Black River introduced a unique service that offered a wide range of fruits and vegetables that were available by the piece and not by a one-case minimum. All the institutional kitchens at which I worked during the 1970s ordered only limited produce amounts that typically included iceberg lettuce, tomatoes, carrots, onions, lemons, and grapefruits.

I have been buying produce from Black River for the last forty years. Since its opening day, the biggest bill that I pay every month to feed the guests at New Life comes from Black River Produce. The second biggest bill I pay every month is to a health food co-op company for healthy grains and other items.

I have witnessed the progressing emphasis on healthy food. In the contemporary health food store, there are so many choices, many of which are more expensive. Learning to navigate a health food store or health food section will teach you that most of the products just have overpriced sugar, fat, and salt while usually having less chemicals added. I will talk about this phenomenon more in the health food section.

The third biggest bill is for commercial food and comes from an institutional food distributer. I would venture to say that any restaurant, including all the ones I have ever worked in and you have gone to, would not have the New Life purchase food ratio. More likely, a restaurant's biggest purchase amount would come from an institutional food company. When I was a cook, I remember reading a magazine titled *Volume Feeding*.

I always thought that was so funny, realizing we often think more about the volume of food rather than quality and nutrition.

These purchase ratios will be relevant to your wellness oasis. You'll notice the locations in the grocery store where you spend time and where you select food for purchase. You should also be aware of your choices at health food stores, convenient stores, restaurants, and social events in your life. There will be more about how to do this in later chapters.

During the last forty years, I have dealt with many different food plans and diets, while never changing my New Life food philosophy. At its start, New Life was to be a new life for me, a summer during which, instead of eating unhealthy food in the institutional kitchen's where I had worked, I could prepare healthy food in the New Life kitchen and provide for myself and the guests, be active, and heal myself and others.

I chose to change my environment to change my health. You will not have to start your own business to do the same. Once you see the underlying principles involved, you will be able to customize and continually refine your approach. Eventually, you will be living a new life without thinking about it so much. The key to this transformation is to get beyond thinking about it and rather simply practice and live the lifestyle.

When I lecture, I do a little dieting trivia and ask, for example, which diet advocated that you eat large amounts of animal fat but prohibited you from eating a tomato. Then I ask about the one where you were only allowed fruit until noon and prohibited eating a potato whenever you were eating chicken. I then would ask guests to think of themselves as the managers of a produce section in the grocery store. Suddenly, the only thing people wanted was grapefruit. Like so many diets the "grapefruit diet" was one of many fad diets. Over time this lecture came to be called "Decades of Dieting Insanity."

I had to deal with all these different diets that people wanted to serve as their magic bullets. But I have maintained the same food philosophy since the day New Life opened with the message "diets do not work." If a diet appears to be working for you, it's because you are not eating the foods or nonfoods that made you feel that the diet was the solution in the first place. The diet is short term. You want to be done with it as soon as possible. It is like holding your breath for a week. The benefits are short term. There is little left in place as a foundation for long-term changes. Your thinking has not changed. Your environment is the same. Your behavior has not changed. You will remember that I have termed this and continue to refer to it as "institutional dieting."

Who Was Nathan Pritikin?

Nathan Pritikin became my hero. He was a wealthy inventor with many credited patents. He was diagnosed with a heart condition in 1957 and began to do extensive research on his situation. Unlike anything I could hope to do at that time, he examined eating habits scientifically. In the mid-1970s, he developed an institute in California, where a person could go to his twenty-eight-day retreat. His staff of doctors and research scientists did blood work to create a complete diagnostic workup while examining a participant's personal lifestyle. He and his team wanted to prove scientifically that what you ate could heal your body.

A salad bar of fruits and vegetables and some whole grains combined with a small amount of animal protein was the institute's residents' main fare, and fat was almost totally eliminated. This concept became the foundation of the New Life cuisine.

Through research and the assessment of the diagnostic workup before and after his program, he proved that what one eats and continued eating matters. Pritikin had sound science behind his claims. In his program he also had guests exercise by walking up and down the beach. Many of his residents who came to the institute and were hardly able to walk in the front door on their own were jogging along the beach twenty-eight days later.

When Pritikin first started making these claims, his work was extremely controversial. I have seen television interviews with him during which his findings were very much disputed and dismissed as scientifically unproven. When Pritikin died, his *New York Times* obituary called him the most profound nutritional thinker of the twentieth century.

The Pritikin approach taught me so much and validated what I was trying to do. I wanted to reach potential guests who wanted to get healthier so they wouldn't find themselves in life-threatening situations like Pritikin's early guests. This is what my life's work, New Life and *authentic wellness*, is all about.

I developed what I called a modified Pritikin plan. I continued to modify the cooking over the years and made a cuisine that resembled Pritikin's, but my adaptation had enough food to accommodate a lot of exercise. In doing this, I sought to demonstrate how we can modify our food environment. The means to modify your food environment involved a completely different approach to eating that limits nonfood and prescriptive dieting relationships with food. *Authentic wellness* involves the creation of a new paradigm for every aspect of your twenty-first-century relationship with your food, fitness practices, and wellness environment. Calorie counting, dieting, or the body mass index, scales, and measuring will not enter our discussion. We will talk about *real* water-based food with positive health attributes.

There will be some recipes. The recipes presented will outline the practical means that may assist you in your lifestyle adjustments and support your desired food-related behaviors. This book aims to change your perspective on the food you eat. You will create a personal and subjective relationship with food that will allow your water-based body to function in a manner that initiates and achieves *authentic wellness*.

A Historical Perspective on Our Relationship with Food

In college I read a book published in 1970 titled *Future Shock* by Alvin Toffler, which sold more than five million copies. Toffler pointed out that since my birth in 1950, change has occurred in an exponential rate never experienced in human history. He examined this change and how it has affected every aspect of our lives. This book had a powerful impact on me.

In 1970 while I was going to college at Florida State University, I worked an overnight shift at the computer lab. This computer was housed in a large basement-size air-conditioned room. I fed the data cards into the computer for processing. In my fourth year of running New Life, I bought an Apple computer that I put on a desk, spending much time during the off-season learning how to use it. Today I have a smart phone. I can be anywhere and take reservations and do research for this book while holding the phone in my hand. That is future shock.

We have come so far in technological and social transformation just as Toffler talked about in his book, all having positive and negative ramifications. But because of the food we eat and the sedentary lifestyle that has been developed since the mid-twentieth century, we have made limited positive changes in our relationship with food. This has created significant negative health benefits. This book will address these negative consequences not so much as a societal issue but as a subjective and personal issue that we can each address with a transformation of our relationship with our bodies and minds to then establish *authentic wellness*.

Using nutritional coaching, I have designed a completely different measure of how the food you eat affects your body and mind. To grasp this, you must understand what your body is and realize how almost all the information that you know has flowed from the promotion of institutional dieting. To move away from the promotional clutches of institutional dieting, you must learn to disperse change across the many different dimensions through which *authentic wellness* may be attained.

As you begin this journey, remember that I have tried to organize this book into sections, but the separations are artificial and academic. The education, sociology, and psychology of eating all overlap in many overt and subtle ways. We can define the body and mind as separate categories, but our living reality informs us of their connections. I had to find my own path, and you can read about that in the biography; however, that's what led me to this multidimensional approach. Your path to *authentic wellness* will be discovered and hastened by a deeper understanding of the many dimensions of your relationship with food.

Let's Begin This Reeducation

Eating is universal to all human beings. We must eat. The makeup of the human body is also universal. The truth is that our body is about 65 percent water. It would make sense to eat foods that are water-based. This is true for everyone reading this book, whether you are rich or poor, tall or short. Whatever age or gender, we are all mostly water. All living things are water-based.

I once discussed this reality with one of my favorite body workers. She used the metaphor of a swamp to describe our bodies—mostly water with all kinds of other living things suspended in a swampy environment. I like to think of us as a pond. If the water in the pond is overwhelmed with pollution, the pond's ecology loses its health over time. We have all heard the expression "You are what you eat."

Consider the characteristics of our relationship with food prior to 1950. The vast majority of the food eaten was water-based, unprocessed, unpackaged, and pretty much based on the seasons. Consequently, prior to 1950, the human relationship with food was water-based, and the human body was comprised of approximately 65 percent water.

The times before 1950 are not presented for consideration to romanticize them. Our pre-1950 relationship with food did not lack its own nutritional tragedies—famine, scurvy, poverty, and other causes. Today we have too much nonfood. As in the case of our relationship with technology prior to 1950, our relationship with food also changed at a rather slow pace.

The post-1950 period has witnessed unprecedented changes in our relationship with food. Over time the composition of our bodies has transformed. We are no longer water-based beings. Our bodies are a muddle of water, fat, and chemicals. Look at yourself and the people around you at work, the amusement park, sporting events, and where you shop. Look at your neighbors and family members. If you listen to the news, you'll hear about the alarming rates of obesity and degenerative diseases. Look at pictures of people before and after 1950 and notice how our girth has grown dramatically.

The Food-Industrial Complex, Big Pharma, and Institutional Dieting

The food-industrial complex is the vast cluster of food production and manufacturing interests and enterprises. These entities govern every aspect of our food—seed, cultivation, harvest, transport for processing and packaging, storage, transport, and public sale. This is a far cry from the days when most people lived on farms. The food-industrial complex continues to respond to the popular preferences for food convenience and palatability that arose in the 1950s. The complex has done so by incorporating excessive sugar, fat, salt, and chemicals, all of which have moved our food substance increasingly away from its primary basis in water. These kinds of foods compose what I call *nonfood*, and they have dramatically overwhelmed our food supply.

Big Pharma is the collective domination by large pharmaceutical corporations over the choice and priority of scientific research required for the development, clinical testing, and marketing of drugs that are needed to accommodate our changed body composition. I am sure you notice that there are so many commercials about drugs, and there are very few about water-based foods like apples and avocados. Big Pharma relentlessly peddles us on the expectation that the drugs they produce will be effective in addressing obesity and other negative health issues related to the food we eat and prevalence of a more sedentary lifestyle. The drugs provide additional chemicals intended to counteract the negative effects of ingesting high volumes of sugar, fat, and salt. We will go into this in more detail. These added chemicals have further unhealthy ramifications and side effects. This cycle continues, and as mentioned, it is accelerating.

The influences of institutional dieting or going on a diet perpetuate the belief that a directed linear regimen of eating less food or only particular kinds of food for a limited period will result in weight loss. This is a one-size-fits-all approach. In targeting weight reduction and control, institutional dieting encourages the illusion that time and food specifications are measures adequate to restructure complex, multidimensional, food-related behaviors. I have dealt with institutional dieting since the day New Life opened. As I have said, I have kept the same New Life food philosophy, and I have always felt that it was all about lifestyle change. Patience, some good guidance, and a transitional period will equip you to replace the indoctrination you have received through your institutional dieting experiences. You will learn to recast your interactions with food. This will improve the water purity of the pond that is your body and the source of your well-being and *authentic wellness*. The goal is to move away from the one-size-fits-all institutional dieting approach.

You Are the Focus

The array of these three institutional giants entrenched against the prospects of any alternative vision's success is daunting. Yet there are alternatives that I wish to propose in this book. My alternatives will be scientifically informed, personalized to your lifestyle, and derived from forty years as a professional practitioner in nutrition and fitness and how the body and mind are connected.

A dear friend of mine named Lee Jacobs died in peaceful sleep at the age of ninety-two in 2014. Lee came of age in the America that existed well before the 1950 threshold that divided our food supply off from the water-based authenticity prior to that point. Lee was a most gentle man. He had served as bomber pilot over Europe in World War II. He practiced yoga and meditation in his continuous desire for personal growth and self-improvement.

Lee taught me a lot. His insights came in depression experiences he related to me as well as such practicalities as his advice to chew each mouthful of food at least twenty times. In what turned out to be the final week of his life, he answered a question I put to him about the secret of meditation or prayer. His response was "to listen." He believed that listening should be experienced as an active process—a verb rather than a noun.

Lee's wisdom about listening will be useful as you begin to encounter the nonlinear and subjective approach to your food relationship and food behaviors. It will sharpen your awareness of how your food makes your body feel. It will allow you to recognize your body as it is when it is genuinely hungry. It will clarify your experience of that spike in blood sugar levels that follows immediately after that candy bar's simple carbohydrates enter the bloodstream. It will furnish you with a sensory grasp of the difference between that sugar rush and the absorption of complex carbohydrates. These forms of listening will run this "body talk" through your mind. New pathways between your senses and your cognition will share the back-and-forth essence that is the mind-body connection, which is so critical to nurturing the process of personal transition that's under way. You will look and feel better.

Science, reason, and my lifetime devotion to personal growth are on our side. Well-being will not just be an objective of *authentic wellness*. It will be the means, the practice, and the process. You will benefit both immediately and over the course of your lifetime. You will do so on a personal and gradual basis. Your lifestyle will shape your choices. You will not be directed or restricted. You will be encouraged to experiment and refine your practice.

So let's get started!

CHAPTER 2

The Education

I Will Be Your Guide

We will now look at ways to change your food life based on my forty years of learning, observation, experimentation, discovery, and practice. Your age, size of family, food budget, work, cooking habits, and understanding of the food available in your life will all play a role in your own *authentic wellness* and a healthy body and mind.

This section will acquaint you with ways you can move gradually and progressively away from the present structure of your food life. It is personal to you, not a one-size-fits-all institutional diet. Any sport or education pursuit requires training. Institutional dieting doesn't require training. *Authentic wellness* does. I want to suggest measures and experiences that maximize prospects for change that's compatible with the lifestyle you have and with the lifestyle that emerges. That is why this is about training and not about dieting. A new blueprint will provide you with a sense of your relationship with food in the twenty-first century.

If you read the biography section, you will learn that my life built upon the opportunity that presented itself for me to leave my institutional kitchen environment. Life in that environment was no longer acceptable. I had to learn a whole new way of approaching my relationship with food. It didn't include institutional dieting. For most of you, it will be about letting go and relearning outside institutional dieting.

Where you begin your *authentic wellness* is personal, unique, and specific to you alone. You must recognize that the process of change as it relates to food and fitness in your life is yours alone to discover and to achieve. Most of you have been "struggling with your weight." You have realized that dieting has not worked. Therefore, you are ready to approach eating and wellness strategy using a different perspective. A different course requires a mind-set change when it comes to your relationship with food.

I have seen New Life guests begin to let go of institutional dieting and embrace a multidimensional approach to how they eat. The scale, calories, and dieting lose relevance as people come to understand their relationship between the food they eat and the effects on their appearance, how they feel, and illnesses like high blood pressure, adult diabetes, and cardiovascular disease. For example, I think one of the best indicators of your overall health as you age is not weight but how much medication you are taking and your blood pressure. We don't know what we would be in a healthy, water-based body in the twenty-first century. Some people think they should look and weigh what they were when they were younger. Others might like how they look after a diet and then gain all the weight back and add even more. We have not defined what a true twenty-first-century body is supposed to be like. But we do know that something is wrong and that what we are doing is not working.

Since I was born, the grocery store has dominated our relationship with food. It has changed dramatically since I started New Life forty years ago. What is truly amazing to me is that regardless of where you live and shop, the configuration, design, and inventory of stores is almost the same and seems to maximize and encourage your purchase and consumption of products that contain the sugar, fat, salt, and chemicals that deny us the water-based *real* foods we require.

Think about all the ads you see for sugary, fatty, and salty products and then the ads about medications used to deal with the effects of sugar, fat, and salt. These cost billions of dollars. It must be working, or it would not be happening. That is the environment you are dealing with. I have rarely if ever seen an ad for a banana, orange, avocado, or eggs. The ads for medication should scare you enough to get on an *authentic wellness* path.

From the most fundamental standpoint, I want to be the guide who walks with you as you encounter anew the understanding and selection of your food in an *authentic wellness* mind frame. This guidance and your experience are fundamental but not absolute. The experience is subjective. It will become yours alone. There is no absolute right or wrong method or routine. After your initial guidance, your shopping will begin to gear itself to your specific personal journey. Once on your own, it would, in fact, be natural for your experiences to change depending on your personal circumstances. There's no reason to be hard on yourself about any of this process.

You will become a much more educated consumer, and as you change, you will notice new products and food choices. You will react to your food environment with different emotional impulses. The way that you feel about your food will change to create a foundation for your experience of *authentic wellness*. The ongoing outcome will yield a home environment that conforms to and promotes food that tastes good, is convenient, and fits your budget, creating a healthy lifestyle.

You will add to what you know about preparation in a manner that is appropriate to your cooking skills, the preparation time you have available, the convenience you require, your taste preferences, the size of your household, and your household's economy. Almost immediately, your efforts will promote your sense of well-being. And after that, you will adapt the practices and pace of your transition to a lifestyle supportive of *authentic wellness*.

What Real Food Is

Real food is water-based food. It is healthy for you because eating real food adds to the purity of the pond that constitutes your body. Ideally, real food is the only food that you should eat. Eating nonfood reduces the purity of your pond and increases your girth and the likelihood of contracting a degenerative disease. Eating only real food is not the goal. The goal is to understand the value of water-based food and evolve toward having more of it. As you do, you will change.

A good overview of real food is provided by *The 150 Healthiest Foods on Earth* by Jonny Bowden. This is a great source for identifying these foods, all of which are, of course, water-based. The book also provides an authoritative understanding of these foods' positive benefits, including their antioxidant, anti-inflammatory, and probiotic properties. It is also interesting to read about the nutritional micro and macro values of these foods. Most importantly, these foods will all have positive effects on one's health. These are the basic foods that you find in the produce and peripheral sections of the grocery store.

Interestingly, Bowden does not include wheat among the 150 real foods cited. This omission was, no doubt, intentional. This is because in my opinion almost all wheat grain products contain enriched flour. Check this out during your grocery store tour. But there are wheat options that are totally wheat. The visual included in this chapter depicts a whole grain wheat *berry*.

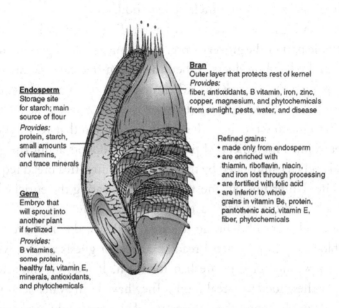

Endosperm
Storage site
for starch; main
source of flour
Provides:
protein, starch,
small amounts
of vitamins,
and trace minerals

Germ
Embryo that
will sprout into
another plant
if fertilized
Provides:
B vitamins,
some protein,
healthy fat, vitamin E,
minerals, antioxidants,
and phytochemicals

Bran
Outer layer that protects rest of kernel
Provides:
fiber, antioxidants, B vitamin, iron, zinc,
copper, magnesium, and phytochemicals
from sunlight, pests, water, and disease

Refined grains:
• made only from endosperm
• are enriched with
  thiamin, riboflavin, niacin,
  and iron lost through processing
• are fortified with folic acid
• are inferior to whole
  grains in vitamin B6, protein,
  pantothenic acid, vitamin E,
  fiber, phytochemicals

In recent times, the portions of the berry termed the bran and the germ have been removed from the berry. The bran was removed for cosmetic reasons. Wheat germ was taken out because the germ has a fat content of about 10 percent, which affects the shelf life of the wheat. To better preserve the product's shelf life, *enriched* flour was developed. Many of the wheat's natural ingredients were replaced with other ingredients of less nutritional value. The enriched claim sounds good, but it is not.

The transition of a real food (in the form of the whole grain wheat berry) into a nonfood is complete. As manufacturers compete for their share of the consumer market, similar efficiencies are sought and applied to products that were once real food and have been transformed into nonfood. As manufactures of these products are beginning to understand your demands for more natural products, you must remember that the only wheat that is whole wheat has the whole berry of the wheat. The word natural means nothing at it relates to what you read on the front of a food product. Even if 100 percent whole wheat is indicated, make sure you are aware of the other ingredients added, in particular sugar, to the product that will reduce the nutritional value. The only true 100 percent wheat products that I have found must be bought in the frozen section of the grocery store. Careful scrutiny of the ingredients on the label will increase the likelihood that you will purchase real food.

In my view, just about everybody has an allergy to the wheat products in the middle part of the grocery store, including all baked goods, cookies, crackers, and related products. When the gluten-free craze came to New Life a few years ago, it was overwhelming how many people said they didn't want the 100 percent whole wheat products served at New Life. They wanted me to serve them the gluten-free option that very frequently contained refined ingredients. I persisted in my doubts about the gluten-free trend and feel vindicated by the reduction gluten-free bread requested at New Life. Unfortunately, most went back to eating the enriched flour so much a part of the middle part of the grocery store.

Another element of defining real food is that it doesn't have a label. It truly blows my mind when I read an article or guests ask me whether avocados, raw nuts, or eggs are bad for them. It really is important to realize that these foods are real foods. They have been available as staples of the food supply before the dominance of the food-industrial complex. To be concerned that an avocado may be high in fat is silly. Nobody has clogged arteries from eating too many avocado, nuts, and eggs. These are all real foods.

In learning about real food, understand they all have a high-water content. For example, meat has about 50 to 70 percent water, although it has been considered not good for your pond. Eggs are one of nature's most nutritional powerhouses. Unless your medical professional cautions you otherwise or you have eating restrictions self-imposed for a variety of reasons, meats and eggs can be versatile menu items. Of course, fish makes the team as well. In any case, with the possible exceptions noted, please attempt to include meats and eggs in your food plans. Purchase the best quality of these you can afford. If you are a vegetarian, then be sure to learn about real foods that will satisfy your protein needs.

The Grocery Store

Your education can now continue with visits to a grocery store. Your experience will resemble most closely a visit to a museum. The first such visit to a typical chain grocery store should take about an hour. You are not there to purchase anything but merely to stroll up and down the aisles to note the layout and get familiar with label reading. When you visit again, your shopping experience will be completely new.

During your first visit, start with the produce section, which is usually found on the right side of the store. Notice that none of these foods have labels. They are real water-based foods that you should buy. As you complete your stroll, note the time you spent in this section. Most of New Life's food budget is spent on items from the produce section. This was not the case when I helped with the ordering in any institutional kitchen as a professional cook. I would guess that almost every restaurant does not have produce as its biggest expense. The produce area is where you will eventually spend most time in your shopping experience.

Continue to the typically vast area that comprises the middle aisles of the store. Although about 80 to 90 percent of the middle portion of the store did not exist in the mid-twentieth century, the products here have come to eclipse and dominate everything else offered in food stores. The products in this section of the store are not healing foods. Nevertheless, these products are a gargantuan portion of our food culture and are backed by billions of dollars in advertising. The domination of food culture by these products assures that most grocery stores will turn into universal replicas of one another. That is why there is such an increase in girth circumference and degenerative health issues. I have shopped in grocery stores in many parts of the country, and I am so amazed how similar they are.

Check out the rows and rows of cookies, crackers, chips, breads, candies, and of course, all the sodas and sugary drinks. These foods are selling, or they would not be in the store. Spend time going to the products that you buy in this section. Think about why you buy them. Feel the tasty and emotional attachment you have to these foods. Notice the vast array of colorful packaging with all the claims these products make. You'll see words like "all natural," "high fiber," or "low fat." But as you will learn from label reading, most ingredients in these products are sugar, fat, salt, chemicals, and a wide range of other substances unrecognizable to you. These products are not good for your pond. Again, please approach this environment's different sections as if you were moving among the different galleries in a museum. Try to sense how these foods and nonfoods comprise a substantial part of your life. I have learned to skip whole aisles, but when I do look down these aisles, I react viscerally to what this nonfood does to us and to our world. It has to change!

You will learn that label reading is essential. It is the label that matters and not what the front of the box says. The box can claim anything, but the label is what matters. This practice is vital to acquainting you with the vast realm of products that you should avoid. Notice the sea of nonfood. Go and select a few of the items in each section and run your finger over the top of them. Notice that there is no dust on these products. This means that they sell on a regular basis. That frankly blows my mind. Maybe you don't buy all that stuff, but someone does. Your task is navigating through it all to benefit your pond.

You should not purchase products with the following ingredients on their labels: cottonseed oil, palm oil, hydrogenated, dextrose, corn syrup enriched flour, and yellow or some other dye number. Don't or limit buying anything with ingredients you don't understand. If you do decide to buy it, at least you've given yourself the chance to recognize what you're putting in your pond. Cottonseed oil is like eating your shirt!

As you will see, once you resolve to dramatically decrease purchasing products with these ingredients, you will have eliminated about 80 percent of all products located in the food store's middle aisles. At this point, you should also look at food that you really like and have bought at the store on a regular basis. Focus on these items. You might find alternatives that have better ingredients. You could try those. For example, look for a tomato sauce or beets that don't have sugar added. You will also look at nonfood products that you really enjoy. Pick a few, and in the beginning, do not give these up. Remember, this is a nonauthoritarian subjective process. Is sugar or salt your thing? Or both?

The canister of mac and cheese is my favorite example of the value of label reading and not assuming or accepting the claims of products at face value. One would think that the product is simply macaroni and cheese with milk and butter. If so, why are the label's ingredients so extensive?

Another example is peanut butter. Find peanut butter with 100 percent peanuts and no sugar or cottonseed oil. With jams and jelly, is the first ingredient the actual fruit, or is it sugar or corn syrup? You will see all kinds of health claims on the box, but it is the label that you want to understand. Artificial sweeteners have never been included in New Life cuisine and should not be a part of your cuisine either. Over time it would be a good idea to cut down or eliminate these altogether.

Bear in mind these examples of mac and cheese and peanut butter. These foods are universal in the sense that we—especially children—all have these foods to eat at home. We purchase and consume these products pretty much whether we are wealthy or not. Accordingly, we should strive to purchase these products in their real food versions—that is, in those versions that are totally (or as substantially as available) natural and free or extremely limited from sugar, fat, salt, and chemical ingredients.

This is not to minimize the reality that the real food versions of these products are generally more expensive than their nonfood versions. I am familiar with the presumed imperative of purchasing nonfood versions of these products because of poverty. I did not even become aware of the distinction between the commercial peanut butter that I ate as a child and the 100 percent sugar-free, real food version of peanut butter that I discovered as a college student in the co-op operated in the Seventh-day Adventist Church's basement.

Certainly, your economic situation ought not to be the definitive barrier to buying and eating real food. Many real foods like brown rice, even pasta, lentils, canned beans, quinoa, split peas, and garbanzo beans all with a bit of creativity and added vegetables can be made into very economical food that your pond will love. You need a strategy that is also based on the size of your family and how much time you have for the preparation of the food. There are many new products that are coming available. More and more people are looking to change to healthier water based foods. Remember *authentic wellness* is a subjective process of change.

Real food becomes more affordable when you are aware of sales, seasonality, and other purchasing practices. A rice maker, discussed elsewhere, can provide a low-cost and easy-to-use vehicle for considerable economies that allow for the purchase and consumption of real food so that

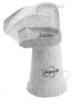

you can cook affordable healthful and delectable meals.

Popcorn : Inexpensive snacks can be healthy. Purchase a jet popcorn cooker. Then look for the one- or two-pound bag of popping corn, usually on a bottom grocery shelf, for a couple of dollars. Adding parmesan cheese, nutritional yeast and olive oil to the popped corn. You do not need to buy any of those microwave popcorn options. Check the ingredients (e.g., cottonseed oil, palm oil, dextrose, etc.). A jet popper creates a wonderful healthy alternative for your pond.

Please continue to the frozen food department. There, you will find ice cream, pizza, and all kinds of frozen, enriched, flour-based products with long lists of ingredients. You will also find frozen fruit and vegetables that might not always be as healthy as fresh fruits and vegetables but do have a place in supporting the well-being of your pond. If a fruit or vegetable is in season, it is always best to get it in the produce section, but during the off-season, the frozen fruit and vegetable is a healthy option. This is an example of where making food choices is not exact.

Most grocery store sections have a so-called "healthy food" section in the freezer area. These can include such healthy ingredient items as 100% whole wheat bread and English muffins, frozen pizza, burritos, and pot pies. Look at the label, and you will notice ingredients that you know the meaning of and that are not dominated by sugar, fat, and salt. They also can serve as quick meals or snacks when you are going to an event that you know will not have healthy food available.

Now go to the far-left side of the store. The dairy and meat locations will usually be different in each store. Find the eggs, yogurt, and cheeses. Find the hot dog and luncheon meat areas too. The hot dogs trigger my recall of a Ralph Nader visit to Florida State University while I was a student there.

In addition to Nader's car safety concerns, his presentation made me fear the nitrates and other pernicious ingredients in hot dogs and luncheon meat. On the streets of New York and at ball games, I have eaten hot dogs. I have never purchased hot dogs or luncheon meat from a grocery store. I do like vegetarian hot dog options in the health food store with the 100 percent whole wheat hot dog buns from the frozen food area. There's not much taste, but it's healthier. I do put ketchup (most have sugar added) and mustard on top. As indicated previously, however, there are special occasions and unique cultural events at which I have made exceptions—even for hot dogs. You should also make exceptions for yourself.

I also can't understand why hot dogs and luncheon meat have sugar and other nonmeat ingredients added. My theory is that sugar is cheaper than pork or other meat ingredients. Sugar is in so many products in so many ways—dextrose, fructose, corn syrup, sugar, and others that look more like chemicals. Did you know that most thanksgiving turkeys have added sugar? Why?

Resume your stroll throughout the store. You may encounter a baked goods area, which you should avoid or buy in a limited manner. The deli and sushi areas might have a few healthy options. Many stores now have a kind of health food section. It might include bulk nuts, grains, and brown rice as well as some food that you usually find in a health food store. Grocery stores are responding to the fact that more and more people do want healthy water-based choices.

Finally, for the conclusion of your first visit, take a mental inventory of how much time you would normally spend in each section of the grocery store and the products you buy. Again, remember this is a personal process of change that will evolve over time.

Your second visit includes actual shopping. This process is the most instructional in your encounter with the many products in the store's middle aisles. Since most of your budget should lean more toward real water-based food, you can skip the snack and candy aisles. If you need the emotional safety of your traditional treats, go ahead and put some candy, cookies or chips in your shopping cart. Although your treats are not water-based foods, the increase in water-based real food you are putting in your pond will better enable your body to handle the effects of the nonfood intake. In the longer term, your need for your traditional treats will subside.

New Life would not purchase any of the middle aisle breads. It's likely that to some degree, most people would be allergic to most of these additive-loaded middle-aisle breads. If you only eat gluten-free items, then you have educated yourself on what your wheat allergy permits you to buy.

Not all products in the frozen section have these kinds of healthy ingredients. That is why you, just as I did, should spend some time learning and reeducating yourself.

These labels are from the English muffin, bread, and tortilla we use at New Life for breakfast, a fresh turkey sandwich and a tortilla lunch. Notice the ingredients. All are real foods with no added sugar. You will find them in the frozen section of health food stores and grocery store healthy food sections.

English Muffin

These unique English muffins are different from any you've ever tasted. Each muffin contains seven gently sprouted, organically grown grains and absolutely no flour. We add just the right amount of malted barley and a pinch of sea salt. Try them served warm to release their rich nutty flavor. With just one bite, you'll know they're a food for life!

Bread

Ingredients: Organic Sprouted Wheat, Filtered Water, Organic Malted Barley, Organic Sprouted Rye, Organic Sprouted Barley, Organic Sprouted Oats, Organic Sprouted Millet, Organic Sprouted Corn, Organic Sprouted Brown Rice, Fresh Yeast, Organic Wheat Gluten, Sea Salt.

Tortilla Wrap

Inspired by the Holy Bible verse "Take also unto thee Wheat and Barley and Beans and Lentils and Millet and Spelt and put them in one vessel and make bread of it" (Ezekiel 4:9).

Ingredients: Organic Sprouted Wheat, Filtered Water, Organic Sesame Seeds, Organic Sprouted Soybeans,, Organic Sprouted Barley, Organic Sprouted Millet, Organic Sprouted Lentils, Organic Sprouted Spelt, Sea Salt.

Please note the water based real ingredients in these products. You know what the ingredients are. They are authentic real food that New Life uses. We only buy breads from the store's frozen foods section.

You will not find this kind of authentic nutritionally food in the middle part of the grocery store. Give it a try. Attempt to pick what you think would be the best three cereals, crackers, and cookie options by finding label ingredients that do not contain cottonseed oil, palm oil, dextrose, corn syrup enriched flour, yellow or some other dye number, or any ingredient you do not recognize or cannot pronounce. You will not find much. If you do put them in your cart.

Here's an interesting experiment. Take a slice of any of these products and put it on a plate in your kitchen. Then take a slice of any bread product from the middle part of the grocery store. Put that on a plate on your countertop. You will notice that in about five to seven days, the products we use will begin to grow mold. The one from the middle part of the grocery store will last for a very long time without mold. That is because it is not real food. All wheat products that don't use the whole wheat berry will not grow mold for a very long time.

It truly is overwhelming. Spend some time looking at the package colors and the box blurbs that make all kind of claims. The boxes might be different, but the ingredients on their labels will be very close or perhaps the same. I remember watching an episode of *The Phil Donahue Show* when he was talking to a corn farmer. Many of you might not remember Phil Donahue. The farmer showed a small bag of corn. He mentioned that the bag held the equivalent of one ear of corn. He then showed a box of cornflakes. It turned out that the box that the cornflakes came in cost more than the amount of corn that was in the box.

Among the canned fruits (among which a few have no sugar added) and vegetable items, the beets are about the only ones that we should consider purchasing. In fact, without much exception, in the store's middle aisles, there are so few ingredients healthy enough to consume that the best advice would be to exclude as many items from this area as possible from your shopping list. However, you do need to spend time looking at these products and making your own decisions.

There are a few exceptions in the middle aisles. I think sardines are a very health food. I like them with the olive oil or mustard. Canned clams add a wonderful addition to pasta with vegetables. Parmesan cheese and a bit of olive oil are wonderful. Pasta is still mostly enriched wheat, but it can be a staple if you have a limited food budget. Adding broccoli, carrots, frozen peas, and any vegetables, prepared or store-bought tomato sauce without sugar, and perhaps some ground beef makes for an authentic and inexpensive meal. Try to choose pasta that is not so white. Check out all the different pasta options. In any one instance, the nutritional value increase is not that much, but every nutritional encounter accumulates in your body over time. I like the pasta that has a bit more protein added.

Most generally, the ingredients in products from the middle aisles include a combination of the sugar, fat, salts, and chemical substances that attract our taste and preserve the product in its originally manufactured condition if possible. The food manufactures have boosted institutional dieting by manufacturing food that reflects the latest dieting trend. When fat was out, they would focus on products that had lot of simple carbohydrates, which meant a lot of sugar. When sugar was out, they would add lots of unhealthy fats. They have always added too much salt. The media would then go along with these fads, and you, the consumer, would be completely confused because you thought that only calories really mattered. A new fad diet would come along, and the cycle would continue. Let's change that cycle and work toward buying and eating more water-based food with real ingredients reflected on the labels.

The effort you make and the time you spend reviewing the labels of these products will, as mentioned briefly regarding your first visit, teach you about ingredients such as enriched flour, palm oil, corn syrup, cottonseed seed oil, and sodium content. Spend some time really trying to learn about what you are eating. I had to do that to start New Life. You can see what is in the products you buy and begin to connect emotionally with the effect their ingredients might have on the purity of your pond.

Canned soups are problematic because their ingredients will generally approach or exceed the daily 2300mg of sodium that you need. Look at the serving in soups to see how much sodium you get in one can. They try to trick you by saying one serving is a half of a cup of soup. Nobody eats half of a cup of soup for a meal. If you add up all the sodium in one can, it will be close to your daily allowance. Then look at other products in the middle part of the grocery store. You'll see how getting to the 2300mg daily requirement doesn't take much. If you have been buying a lot of food from the middle part of the grocery store, you will probably average around 4000mg or more a day, which is a recipe for high blood pressure. As a test, check out the sodium content of any product in any middle aisle of the grocery store. If one serving has a hundred calories, the sodium content should only be 200mg. This is one-to-two ratio. If you just applied this one-to-two ratio of calories to sodium, you would be amazed at how few products you would purchase.

Having talked about the overuse of sodium, it must be understood that most of the salt in these products is refined salt. A great reference to the history and benefits of unrefined salt can be understood by reading *Salt Your Way to Health* by Dr. David Brownstein.

Soups in restaurants are also high in refined sodium. I know. I used to make them. Most of the time, the flavor comes from a jar of what I call *glop*. It is made up of cheap fats and a lot of salt. Every chef I have hired to work at New Life has had to learn a new way of making soup that dramatically cuts down on salt. At first, they have an impulse to add more salt. But over time their taste buds change, and they get it. This is an example of how *authentic wellness* is a process.

Canned beans are among the very few middle aisle products to consider purchasing. If they don't have added sugar, they are fine. Baked beans don't make the team, but black, kidney, red, and garbanzo beans are a few that are on the New Life menu. It is good to run water through the canned beans to get out most of the salt.

The raw bean is better than the canned bean, but it takes a long time to cook. In this case, I feel that the canned is fine. This is another example of making your own food choices based on health, convenience, cost, and taste.

For drinks, it really comes down to water or seltzer water. Add a lemon or lime. All these new flavored waters are another version of soda. If the drink has sugar, it has a lot. It is better to have the orange rather than orange juice, and most other fruit juices have sugar added. Read the label. There are a few new juice options that have juiced vegetables. I approve of those. I do think some of the new drinks that have a healthful ingredient mix are fine for a quick snack. But the label will tell you that the first ingredient is usually apple or grape juice. My favorite, although sometimes hard to find, is carrot juice. Read the labels and get a sense of what is going on. Remember that classic soda has about ten teaspoons of pure refined sugar. Also, as I will mention over and over, sugar is sugar is sugar.

For beer and wine, I use the phrase "things in moderation." If you have dramatically reduced the chips, enriched flour, crackers, and other items that usually accompany them, then you can have some beer or wine. If you have a drinking problem, that is another issue. One of my favorite drinks is nonalcoholic beer, though it's a bit pricy. There are a lot of different kinds, and they have a great flavor compared to sugar soda and drinks, iced coffee, or tea. I call nonalcoholic beer a malt drink. On a summer day, a cold malt drink is fantastic if it is not a good time to have a regular beer.

In the frozen section, examination of the items will indicate that most of them have ingredients to avoid such as enriched (meaning processed) flour as well as high sodium and sugar content. The fruits and vegetables are the positive exception in the frozen section. These are worth your examination because they can keep you supplied with fruit for shakes and additions to soup. I love to eat frozen cherries as a snack. Let them thaw out a bit before eating. These have no added sugar. I would argue that during the time of year when a fruit or vegetable is out of season, these products are as good or better.

Eggs are a nutritional dream within a food budget, whether you can afford to buy free-range or not. Either way, they are still a nutritional food. It is truly my belief that eggs, yogurt, and cheese are not creating an unhealthy relationship with food either individually or within our society at large. I think it is best to get the plain yogurt and add honey, maple syrup, fresh or frozen fruit, chia seeds, cacao nibs, or other healthy additions. But if you do buy the flavored ones, look at the ingredients carefully. Please let go of the belief that these foods are unhealthy. It is the sugar, fat, salt, and chemicals.

Now let's take a third visit to the food store. On this trip, you'll be doing actual shopping, reading labels as you feel you need to, and staying familiar with the store layout. Your objective will be to invest your time and money in decisions that make the most nutritional sense for you and your household.

For our third visit, let's grab a cart and stop at the produce section in the store. There, you notice that the items on sale include blueberries, grapes, pears, and apples. These fruits are likely on sale because they are in season, fresh, and reasonably priced. It makes sense to buy any that you like and can afford within your budget. I love when fresh cherries are on sale. The produce section also presents vegetables and the building blocks of salad, the gold standard of nutrition. There are also a variety of prewashed salad options in packages. The packaged salads might not be as hefty a portion as a fresh head of red lettuce, romaine, or spinach would be, but these are a good start in any event.

Among the individual vegetable items, the selection is extensive and may include avocados, tomatoes, broccoli, red cabbage, radishes, sprouts, cucumbers, mushrooms, and snow peas. Most of these can be used in a stir fry as well as a fresh salad. You should decide how much to buy based on the size of your household. Because vegetables do not last as long as processed products, you would be wise to get a sense of what you need. I like already cut vegetables for a stir fry. There does seem to be a positive trend toward offering more convenient ways of buying vegetables. This is a good thing. In subsequent trips to the store, you will become adept at determining your produce choices and amounts you need.

At home in addition to fresh salads, you will learn to use some of these items with a simple stir fry or perhaps steamed or cooked in your breakfast eggs. These preparations are examples of *healing* foods. Although you may be understandably uncomfortable with the preparations or the tastes in the beginning, you may also find that the challenge and the adventure will become appealing and even rewarding. If you cook, you can use your recipes in a modified way. If you don't cook, see the section on cooking.

You should not overlook the dressing for your salad. Like most of the other products you have purchased in the past, you have purchased these items from the middle aisles of the food store. As with many other products from the middle aisle, there is a reservoir of tastes and accompanying emotions attached to these items. Like old habits, taste and the emotions attached to them die hard.

Although dressings from the middle aisle will likely require refrigeration after opening, the refrigerated section of the store may be a source of acceptable dressing selections. In applying the dressing, just enough to coat the salad will be sufficient. Learn to enjoy the taste of the vegetables. They do not taste like sugar, fat, and salt, but they can taste good with limited use of a favorite dressing. Keep reducing the amount of dressing until you find the right balance. This will help change your taste buds.

Even though you may be hesitant or the members of your household may not be supportive, begin the process of transitioning to healthy dressings. Try to find dressings that have words you recognize on the label. They will have sugar, fat, and salt, but they are a condiment to your salad. As mentioned, during your store visits, there are many options with which to supplement salads that would maintain a degree of familiarity for your household's salad eaters. Although you can use anything that is *real* food in salads, some suggestions for supplements include meat, poultry, seafood, cheeses, eggs, nuts, seeds, and fruit. There are many salad recipes in cookbooks, magazines, and on the internet. Throw healthy things in. Be creative. Have fun and nurture your pond.

Salads are so primary for proper nutrition and health that it is difficult to overstate how vital they are. Salads are essential, water-based, *real* food. As stated earlier, Pritikin used the true salad bar as his foundation for healing the participants in his program. Each salad should have a wide variety of vegetables, not the restaurant kind with iceberg lettuce, a tomato wedge, two crotons, and large amounts of blue cheese dressing. Recommend items for the base of your salad are mixed greens, spinach, Boston lettuce, kale, and red cabbage.

By the way, sometimes when I feel it is too much of a bother to cook, I go out to eat. If the menu seems to have a good supply of vegetables, I will ask the server to bring me a salad with every vegetable they have in the kitchen, and I will pay extra for the dish. They have never turned me down. I always ask for dressing on the side.

Preparation and consumption of the produce that comprise salads are the first and most important step to restoring our bodies to their basis in water. Salads are our gateway food to *authentic wellness*. With the wide range of vegetable options, you can make salads conveniently and often with a wide range of different vegetables and ingredients. They are great for singles and large families, and you will be amazed how easily they fit into any budget.

Before veering from our discussion of vegetables, we should review some considerations in their use for stir fry meals. Stir fries are strategic meals that make for excellent and nutritious lunches or dinners. So too, the leftover stir fry, either planned or incidental, can become a supplement to another meal with a bit of imagination.

Let's stir fry. Add sliced onions into the frying pan (or wok) with olive oil. Sprinkle in a bit of tamari or soy sauce. You may add your choice of poultry, fish, or beef with fresh garlic that you cut. Then add your vegetables. Add some fresh herbs and maybe a bit of red or white wine. The vegetables may even be precut and prepackaged, or you can obtain them from your food store's salad bar. The following day, you can use a rice cooker to prepare a casserole too. With fresh spinach and the leftovers, you can make a delectable meal. In this way, you can see that beyond its nutritional benefits, the leftover stir fry creates added value as a, time-saving supplement for another meal. You can add nuts and seeds to your stir fry. It's best if you can get these in a health food store or big discount store. It's best to buy raw to avoid added salt and sugar. It is amazing what the labels show that has been added to a basic nut. The sugar, fat, and salt is cheaper than a nut, which means you get less nut for your money when they're sold by weight.

A closer focus on fruit encourages us to find what's on sale and/or what we can afford. On sale or not, I always look for blueberries, raspberries, and strawberries. If I can't get them at a sale price, I still buy as much as I can on my food budget. When I have these berries at home, I have the flexibility to use them sparingly or abundantly with yogurt or cereal or alone as a snack. Have apples, bananas, pears, oranges, or other fruit that can be readily grabbed for snacking. It's great to have a fruit bowl around too. These fruits can be consumed as frequently as possible whenever you're on the run. Fruit is a real, restorative, and healing food that's essential to *authentic wellness*.

Fruit has received two bad raps. One is that they are high in sugar. *So what!* You all have heard this claim. But when have you heard any claim that large segments of the population are experiencing obesity or degenerative disease from eating too much fruit? Your pond loves fruit. It has a lot of water and a lot of the micronutrients that your pond thrives on. You don't have to understand this. Just know that they do, and the processed nonfood in the middle part of the grocery does not. What also is amazing to me is that you don't hear as much about the high sugar content of cookies, cakes, and other high sugar treats.

Fruit also has a bad rap because of pesticides. I did a bit of research about this. Of course, you should wash your fruit. Even washed fruit will retain traces of chemical preservatives. Still, even if you eat a lot of fruit, the effect of any of the chemicals is less unsafe than that of the sugar, fat, salt, and other chemical in the vast majority of food products available. If you have the room in your budget to buy organic, by all means do. Regardless, fruit is paramount to the health of your pond.

I could make an argument that nothing in our food supply is worth eating and that you should just grow your own food and only eat that. At this point in our development, this is not possible. *Authentic wellness* is about the best options within our food supply in the twenty-first century. These are your choices to make.

Because produce is perishable, a good rule of thumb is to plan to use produce within four to five days. At New Life, we receive three to four deliveries of produce each week. Of course, our order consists of about forty different produce items. But in your home, you will likely not be able to use that volume of variety. Instead you can stick to the favorites you come to identify over time. I encourage you to try out unfamiliar produce. Look to see if certain produce is on sale. You may want to try a star fruit, a mango, some kale, or fresh herbs. Of course, the internet can instantly inform you about produce items, how to select the ripest or otherwise best condition, their seasons, a reasonable cost range, and even recipes that contain the items. You can google the item while you are in the produce section!

Among the fruit options, bananas, watermelons, and cantaloupes make up what I call "foundation fruits." They deserve a special tribute because of their value and flexibility. Watermelons cost around $6.00 to $10.00 and can last for days, fortifying your body with water and nutrients. If you are single, just buy a quarter or half melon. Cantaloupes are good to have too. Try to buy them on sale. Sometimes you get them when they're not so ripe. Try to feel them and get the sense of when they will be ready. Bananas are a good value, and you can use them in so many ways.

The advantages of bananas, watermelons, and cantaloupes are substantial. Watermelon and bananas are foods that you can eat to fill up a bit before dining at a restaurant, attending a special event, or even going food shopping. Bananas should be selected when they are ripe to maximize the available vitamins and minerals that accompany their sweetness. If you buy them when they are not ripe, you can just wait for them to ripen. Have bananas around at different stages of ripeness. If they get too ripe, freeze them and use them in a shake. So too, both watermelons and bananas contain extensive nutritional benefits. Your knowledge of these benefits is perhaps less important than your actual eating these fruits. Just get them into your body. Please get out of the institutional dieting framework and stop being concerned about the so-called high calories and sugar content in these foods. These foods have nothing to do with an increase in your girth or the onset of degenerative diseases.

Remember, eating too much fruit is not the issue. The assertion that bananas are fattening and contain too much sugar is a fallacy. Bananas contain 71 percent water. Watermelons contain 91 percent water. Avocados contain 73 percent water. Potatoes contain 70 percent water. Even eggs have 75 percent water. Processed nonfood has zero water.

As you can see, all produce is extremely high in water and nutrition. No one develops health issues from eating avocados, beets, watermelons, bananas, or carrots. It is amazing to me how water-based produce many times will receive bad press but processed food doesn't. Why is this? The sugar or fat content in any of this produce pales in comparison to the nutrition they provide and the fact that they are *real* food comprised primarily of water. Eat as much produce as you want. Use your experience in eating the widest variety possible to develop your taste buds and to expand your nutrition horizon. This is the safest and most important adventure you will ever have, and your appetite will change over time.

Find produce that you like to eat. So too, if you learn—and I mean this—to eat it, you will learn to enjoy it. At the other extreme, if you are hungry, you can pig out on fruit and vegetables. Unlike with ice cream, cookies, candy, or chips, an increase in girth circumference from pigging out on produce is not the issue. We will talk more about pig-out foods later.

If you read on the internet or in the media that fruit and vegetables have any unhealthy calms, including potatoes and sweet potatoes, delete it and move on. Please understand that the unhealthy food issues in our culture have *nothing* to do with the produce section of the grocery store! *Nothing!*

The Health Food Store

In college, I remember visiting the Seventh-day Adventist Church basement to buy foods like 100 percent whole wheat flour, peanut butter without sugar, granola (does have a lot of added sugar), brown rice, and a few other healthy choices. Everything was in big bags or jars, and you put things in your personal containers. They were called food co-ops.

When I started New Life, these co-ops had developed into what became local health food stores. I had to learn about products that would fit into the food I wanted to serve at New Life. I went through the health food store and came up with my own personal strategy for myself and New Life —that is, healthy food items based on convenience, taste, and cost. You will be very amazed by what you read on the labels at the health food store compared to the grocery store. You will not see cottonseed oil, corn syrup, and enriched floor. Yes, a frozen pot pie might cost more in the health food store, but the ingredients are for sure worth the cost. Plus, if more and more of you buy these products, the costs will go down.

In the present day, these health foods stores have evolved into several different kinds of venues, depending on the size of your community. Many towns have health food stores that are privately owned. Other bigger cities have the corporate giant Whole Foods. Like touring a grocery store, you need to spend time in a health food store and look at the packaging and the labeling to learn what is in these so-called heathier foods. You will learn as I did that most of the packaged food has sugar, fat, and salt, though it is a better quality. But is it worth the extra expense. That is your choice based mostly on your budget.

Because people are getting more into health, grocery stores are stocking the products that are in a health food store. They are doing this in two ways. Most grocery stores have a section set aside for these kinds of food. When you learn about them, you will start to notice them in the grocery store. A store may also have these products mixed into the same kind of foods within the store.

You need to find out what health food environment you have in your community and tour the stores just as you did the grocery store. Try a lot of these foods. Some you will like, and some you will not. When I started New Life, carob was very popular. I tried making a carob dessert. In my opinion (and from comments from the guests), carob tasted like dirt. It didn't work for me, so I tried something else. If guests didn't like the food or it was too expensive, I would not have stayed in business. Health food has evolved, and it is my hope that someday the grocery store will become an overall healthy food environment because you have educated yourself on what real food is, and that will affect the food that companies produce. Work toward being a more educated consumer of what you put in your pond.

The Convenience Stores

In the summer of 1972, after I graduated from Florida State, I lived in the suburbs of Atlanta, Georgia, until I could move north to look for a teaching job. I found a job driving a milk truck for a rather large company that delivered milk and dairy products around the newly developing suburbs of Atlanta. On my route I would deliver milk to people's homes. When I would go to work, I would usually see the bigger trucks loading up and getting ready to deliver to the convenience stores. After doing this for a month or so, I was told that the company was going to cancel my route. I worked extra hours closing out these accounts, and as I was doing this, I noticed that convenience stores were popping up in every neighborhood. The big trucks were delivering to those stores, not to the individual homes. This unique situation helped me financially and allowed me to move north.

These convenience stores brought the beginning of concentrated nonfood. I don't remember exactly what was in those stores in those days, but I do know what's in them today. Ironically, I would say that the milk and eggs are about the healthiest items in the stores now.

This is another food environment (actually nonfood environment) where you should spend some time, and you'll see that a convenience store is really the middle part of the grocery store on steroids. When I go in these stores, I feel an emotion from childhood. As well as I can convey it, I am overwhelmed by the presence of the sugar, salt and fat-based nonfood.

On a good day, I'd get a V8, water, or a cup of coffee with a bit of milk and a couple of packets of sugar. Remember, one classic soda has ten to twelve of those packages, and the new sports drinks are not much better. Coconut milk is a pretty good new choice. In some places you can find nuts that don't have added sugar, palm oil, or cotton seed oil. Also, notice how you feel emotionally about this sea of nonfood. You can always choose the apple, orange, or banana, which are usually in a basket in the front part of the store. What is sad is they usually have been there for a while. If you have a healthy shake in your car as you are driving to work or mixed nuts in your pocket or if you come up with some other creative healthy choose, you will be able to avoid these stores other than filling up for gas.

The Institutional Pharmacy

If you need a prescription, you go to a pharmacy. The costs involved nearly defy imagination. Approximately 30 percent of Americans buy high blood pressure medication for almost $50 billion a year. Twenty-nine million Americans with diabetes require medications, glucose-monitoring devices, insulin pumps, and other equipment for a minimum of $1,500 per year, and we also buy countless other drugs for degenerative diseases like heart attacks, strokes, and cancers. Although I would not assert these costs are completely related to the food we eat, I would say that the food we eat are a huge factor.

The next time you pick up your prescription, notice the nonfood products you see as you are walking to the back of the pharmacy. You may be able to buy milk, orange juice, and eggs, but you will otherwise wade into a sea of nonfood that has a significant impact on the purity of your pond. You can't even buy a banana or apple in a pharmacy. Some of these stores have stopped selling cigarettes. But how about stopping the sale of nonfood that has been shown to be a significant factor in the increased need for medications. Take a tour up and down these food aisles. You will be amazed. It might be healthier to pick up your prescriptions in the drive-through.

I can say from talking with guests at New Life during these forty years that many have improved their health by eating real food to the degree that under their health professional's guidance, they have been able to reduce or eliminate medications. Much of the pharmaceuticals available do have tremendous value. It is my belief that the combination of nonfood and prescription drugs housed by the institutional pharmacy is a contradiction that we must address. *Authentic wellness* is a step in the right direction.

Organic and Genetically Modified Organism (GMO)

There is much talk about organic food in comparison to genetically modified foods. My experience has led me to see that neither of these are the absolute solution or problem. They are simply far ends of the spectrum.

I could write a book about how we could consider every food available as bad for any given reason and how you should not eat anything unless you grow it yourself with organic non-GMO seeds in perfect soil and use no pesticides. We do not live in a world where that is possible.

What I have concluded is that yes, organic might be better—if you are willing and can afford to pay extra. But organic or not organic is not the issue. The issue is nonfood with sugar, fat, and salt. As I have said, our pond can handle foods that are water based but not organic. Also, some of the organic labeling frankly is kind of silly. The first time I saw organic maple syrup, I laughed and thought this is just another marketing gimmick. Maple syrup comes from a tree in the woods. If you can afford organic, then buy organic, but as I have said, that is not the issue. The issue is the sugar, fat, and salt polluting our pond.

GMOs are a highly talked about topic. The fact that food companies are buying up seeds and restricting farmers from growing what they want is an important issue. It's important to know what foods have been genetically modified. It is also important to understand the effect of overly aggressive capitalism on certain crops with terminator genes and companies with morally questionable practices. This is an issue we should watch closely, but as a society living in such a system, our goal remains the consumption of mostly water-based foods.

As a kid in the South, I remember how we would get watermelon for cheap, but we didn't eat it in the house because there where so many seeds. We ate watermelon outside and spit out the seeds. Today watermelon has very few seeds. It's more convenient, tastes close to how I remember it, and does have lots of nutrition. We should watch GMOs closely, but it still is not the main issue in our food environment.

Additives in Food

For many years I have talked about additives in food. People are finally saying to me, "If I don't know what it is or can't pronounce it, I try not to buy it." There are so many harmful additives in the grocery products available for purchase that it is always prudent to look up unrecognized ingredients. Do this to assess the pollution that you will be dumping into your pond. A closer look at sodium phosphate would be a valuable illustration of your need to know.

Sodium phosphate, also known as trisodium phosphate or TSP, is a phosphate combined with three sodium atoms. It has many uses today, including toothpastes to whiten and strengthen teeth, although it can also damage teeth. When mixed with water and bleach, it is a common way to clean floors and remove stains. It was also once used as a bowel cleaner in preparation for colonoscopies. When tested, such use was shown to be dangerous because of the effect on the kidneys and renal tract.

Sodium phosphate is used as an emulsifier agent in processed cheese and baked goods. If it was tested among restauranteurs just like the medical community once tested it and the results were published, you would not want it in the food supply along with many other additives.

Sodium phosphate is also an ingredient in a lot of the mac and cheese, which kids eat a lot of. This is just one example of why most additives are not good for your kids or your personal pond. Our foods are flooded with additives that keep drinks from separating and foods from spoiling, and companies also add artificial colors to make a food seem like something it is not.

Vitamins and Dietary Supplements

As a nation, we spend about thirty-five billion dollars on vitamins and dietary supplements. Here is what I think and what I have done. I have taken a multivitamin off and on for many years. I would recommend getting them from a health food store. Some multivitamins have substances added including fruits, vegetables, and other beneficial ingredients. It can get confusing. I would say regardless of which you chose, you will get some health benefit. I don't think; however, you need to take them daily. Maybe even change brands now and then. Multivitamins to me are a food supplement that might or might not have benefits but is worth taking.

Anything beyond a multivitamin is truly perplexing. The abundance of dietary supplements is overwhelming. If you want to spend the time figuring out which ones are beneficial for you personally, go for it. I could have created a New Life vitamin supplement and probably made a lot of money. I don't feel they fit into *Forty Years of Authentic Wellness*, so I have not. The true goal is to get most of your needed nutrients from the food you eat.

Balanced Fitness

In the biography section, I relate my winter spent as a guest of Mel and Enid Zuckerman at the Canyon Ranch Spa in Tucson, Arizona. The inspiration for Canyon Ranch itself was rooted in Mel's experiences at the Oaks Spa in Ojai, California. Mel attributed his recovery from the various health issues that had beset him before his visits to the Oaks. At the Ranch, Mel's recovery displayed itself in his customary morning jog. I ran with Mel just about every morning when I was at the Ranch.

By that time, I was a dedicated runner, and I specialized in the ten-kilometer races. It was my 10K conditioning that got me and Mel through a grueling 26.2-mile Ranch marathon. As we hit the marathon's twenty-mile wall, I recall encouraging Mel to continue the race to its conclusion with a maxim that running more than twenty-six miles a week was unrelated to health. Clearly, Mel's desire to do the first Ranch marathon and my resolve to help him had nothing to do with health. This is nothing against the enjoyment that marathon running brings to so many.

I had learned this maxim and much more during my 1983 enrollment at the Kenneth Cooper Aerobics Institute in Dallas, Texas. There, I became a certified cardiovascular fitness manager. At that time Dr. Kenneth H. Cooper was celebrated as "the father of aerobics." He was the most well-known person to research the benefits of cardiovascular health. In addition to the institute, his influence became global because of his many publications.

During a time when the intense popularity of running arose and the aspiration to run marathons became widespread, the institute taught me the scientific reasoning behind the value of aerobic activity. My own running benefitted from the institute's instruction. I also learned some of the negative aspects of running. A prime example was the institute's maxim that cautioned about the dangers of excess that arose when the underlying motive for fitness activity was not health-related. Cooper said, "If you run more than twenty-six miles a week, you are doing it for something other than your health." My understanding of this principle spurred me to explore the *balance* of health and wellness as it relates to cardiovascular, strength, and flexibility conditioning.

My wellness experience at a yoga retreat and my own practice familiarized me with the benefits of stretching. *Stretching* by Bob Anderson, now in its thirtieth anniversary edition, is a classic book about the subject. I still feel this is the best book about stretching. The historical development of popularized yoga parallels the transition from a work-based lifestyle of the industrial agriculture age to a sedentary lifestyle of the modern metro-digital age that has developed since the mid-twentieth century. Yoga instruction and practice became mainstream in response to the need to maintain the body and muscle flexibility. Yoga became beneficial for our sedentary and overstressed society. The adoption of yoga by the West began in the 1960s and exploded in the 1980s. Hatha yoga has been the most taught and practiced.

The most memorable idea I learned at the six-week yoga teacher training I attended in the summer of 1977 (before I started New Life) was that *age* is chronological but that *aging* should be understood in terms of the spine's flexibility. In our daily routines, we pretty much only use our spine to move or sit in a forward position. Think about it. We sit in cars, chairs, and sofas without much movement. Yoga taught me the many ways our spines can move. This wide range of movement is a genuine path toward body fitness. Try to move your spine in many ways. You will be amazed.

Yoga develops flexibility, strength, body awareness, and balance. The deep breathing routines improve focus and concentration and reduce stress and an accompanying clarity that put you in touch with the mind-body connection. In its original form, the practice extends to yoga's diverse and rich philosophical origins.

Here in America, a competitive, "more is better" zeal expresses itself in various forms of power yoga and other intense yoga workouts. We have taken a soft, relaxing, destressing form of wellness and in many cases made it into an intense form of exercise. When you are looking for yoga in our culture, find a style that fits the body-mind awareness rather than an intense exercise routine. Yoga is truly here to stay, and I recommend it as part of your physical fitness program. At New Life, stretch instruction occurs in classes of Tai Chi, Qi Gong, yoga, and aquatics, all of which are designed for body flexibility.

Strength training should be added to aerobics and flexibility to complete a balanced fitness program for wellness. Strength training has evolved in many ways from a bodybuilding discipline in neighborhood gyms and basements to franchised chains of elaborate fitness centers stocked with rooms full of weight training equipment. At New Life, our daily weight training classes use hand weights to work a great deal on posture and alignment. This is to make sure that as you start to strengthen your body, the process occurs in compatibility with proper body alignment, and balance. A difficulty with intense weight training arises because of the individual's inability to improve strength without impairing body structure. No aspect of a balanced fitness program should be overdone or become a detriment to wellness. When I have visited gyms, it always amazes me to watch people use the weight machines with a complete disregard of their posture, which means that they are developing muscles that are not in alignment with their skeletal structure, which can do damage to all parts of the body.

The fitness revolution that erupted in the early 1980s created many options in attaining fitness for a healthy lifestyle. The inclusion of balanced fitness within a comprehensive wellness program is essential. Some options are better than others. The goal is for you to become an educated wellness consumer.

Balanced fitness involves cardiovascular activity at least twenty or thirty minutes for four or five times a week, strength training about two or three times a week, and stretching and flexibility movement as often as possible. Stretching and flexibility should be highly emphasized. You can stretch any time you want. When I gas up, I will put the pump on automatic and practice standing on one foot. It is amazing to me how someone could go to a yoga class and then drive home with bad posture. Ideally, stretching and increasing flexibility needs to be incorporated into every aspect of your life. Notice ways to improve body alignment and flexibility when you drive, walk, sit, run, do sports, or even how you sleep. You will be amazed at the improvement in your wellness by incorporating stretching and flexibility into your life.

Although the balanced fitness concept did not exist when New Life began, the explosion of fitness information starting in the 1980s has created an overabundances of fitness information. The freedom to experiment and personalize your practice of balanced fitness tilts the odds for success very much in your favor. Walking every day is the simplest way to be active. Enjoy sports like tennis, racket ball, golf, and other indoor and outdoor activities. There is no one true way to accomplish being active, but one discovers, tries, modifies, abandons, and retries many ways. Pick options that are fun and compatible with your lifestyle.

There are many new products and strategies that will help in your fitness quest. The classic suggestions still work. Park your car farther from the store. Instead of the elevator, walk up the stairs in your office. You need to evaluate the available fitness devices in terms of cost, function, convenience, and lifestyle. You can buy a standing desk, a pedometer to count your paces, smart watches, and countless apps. Some of these routines and devices might have value for your *authentic wellness* journey, and others might be just a bunch of junk. Generally, your lifestyle, knowledge level, and the costs are the primary factors in considering your fitness activity and devices. In this way, you are making wellness possible in every present moment. At the same time, the persistence of your practice will reward you with wellness throughout your life. It is wellness of which *you* are the author. It is *authentic wellness*.

CHAPTER 3

The Sociology

The Cocktail Party

Imagine cocktail hour at a wedding reception, office party, or so many other functions where food is the focus. This is an example. You arrive in your best suit or sleek dinner dress and stop at the bar. While the bartender mixes and pours your drink, you grab some nuts from the dish on the bar. This is a fancy party, so these are salted cashews and almonds roasted in oil (maybe even cottonseed oil), and they are probably sugared too. Check out the labels of these products sometime. You munch down about a cup's worth for delivery to your water-based pond.

With drink in hand, you find the hors d'oeuvres. There you look over a variety of cheeses—Brie, Jarlsberg, cheddar, Port Salut, Camembert. These are rich and tasty cheeses. While much to your liking, they average a 70 to 80 percent fat content. You have a sample of each on salted crackers. From the crudité plate, you have a few carrot sticks covered in dip. From the circulating trays, you have a few of the mini sausages, chicken wings, and cheese puffs.

When dinner is announced, you get a refill from the bar and find your place in the dining room. The green salad is drowned in ranch dressing. The entrée is prime rib, green beans almandine bathed in butter or more than likely margarine, and a baked potato with sour cream, butter, and chives. After a momentary hesitation about dessert, you enjoy the generous piece of Bavarian cream pie served with coffee. You cannot forgo the after-dinner drink, a Bailey's port or a Grand Marnier. You must have it all, especially if it is free.

It is possible to get through these events without appearing as a health fanatic and without totally overeating, which is detrimental to your pond. Before the event, you could eat some healthy foods or snacks. Remember the healthy frozen food from the health food or grocery store. Have some in your freezer and use when needed. You could curb your hunger with fruit, vegetables, a whole grain wrap, a sweet potato, or a banana. After arrival, you stand at the bar to order, but your earlier actions allow you to pass on the cheeses. Ordering a Bloody Mary, scotch and soda, or wine allows you to avoid excess sugar and special mixes. Never trust anything with a maraschino cherry!

You go to the crudité table (or other vegetable and fruit area at the party) and stay there. You may eat as much as you want there. Notice how you are feeling during this action. Listen to your reaction to change. Notice how your body feels. Notice if you feel full. What does feeling full feel like? Can you stop when you feel full? These are questions you want to ask in all your eating situations. Even eating the dip is okay because it is better than the cheeses or the hors d'oeuvres. Okay, choose your favorite cheese and have some. I like scallops wrapped in bacon, so I have a few of those. You choose your favorite. I know it is all free, but think about your pond.

At dinner you could request a salad without the bleu cheese. Ask for oil and vinegar if it's available. Unless there is a healthier alternative, perhaps broiled fish, available for the entrée, you could eat some of the prime rib. You should avoid the green beans, which are usually cooked for too long and doused with butter or margarine. Push some of the butter and sour cream aside from the baked potato. Add some pepper or hot sauce. If available, you could try the baked potato with some cottage cheese. You could sample, eat, or avoid the dessert entirely. You could have a drink without any cream after dinner.

The real world doesn't make it convenient for you to eat healthy. The typical cocktail party is a microcosm of the way society is set up for you to eat. Don't be hard on yourself if you find it difficult. It is.

In recent years I have been to events for kids—birthday parties, swim meets, church and school functions. It is amazing to me the domination of sugar, fat, and salt in these situations. Think of what this is doing to children's ponds. However, I will say that when I have tried to point this out, I am called a health nut ruining the fun. This needs to change for the sake of our kids.

Another situation is travel. I spent a winter at Canyon Ranch, a healthy food oasis. Then I traveled back to New Life, another healthy food oasis. I spent four days on highways. The amazing thing was that I couldn't get anything I wanted to eat. I know it's possible to find a grocery store and buy carrots or apples or some healthy option. I didn't want to get off the interstate to look for a grocery store or a decent restaurant. I didn't have the time. I just wanted to go into a highway restaurant and find a healthy meal. It was impossible in the mid-1980s.

Since then, there have been changes. Some of those highway restaurants have salad bars now. Still, though, it's mostly a vast sea of sugar based drinks with islands of hamburgers, pizzas, hot dogs, french fries, and doughnuts. When you're in one of those places, it's hard not to eat the stuff. I think there must be a psychological mechanism that takes effect when you're sitting at a table and see everybody around you having ice cream sundaes. You feel odd, out of place, and out of synch if you order a cantaloupe and cottage cheese. That psychological quirk is a big problem when it comes to dealing with the real world. If you found everyone else in a restaurant ordering healthy and tasty food, you're more likely to do the same.

You should realize that you're bucking the trend, trying to swim upstream when you want to eat healthy foods in most of America. You can begin to change that. Don't be discouraged. Remember that you want to eat mostly water-based food. Do your best. These changes will be different in each situation, creating a process of change.

How Much to Eat

To figure out how much you should eat, you should consider several factors. As we have discussed, we need to change what we are eating by reducing nonfood and supplying water-based foods, whole grains, and real foods. To do this, carrot and celery sticks in the beginning will not cut it. In this respect, you can eat numerous ak-mak crackers (Look these crackers up on the internet. I have been using them for 40 years), apples, and even two or three bananas because over time eating these healthier foods is going to alleviate some of the toxins in your body and help create metabolic change. As you progress, you can add carrot and celery sticks with peanut butter and over time reduce the amount of food you are eating. The most important factor is getting water-based food in your body.

When you are eating water-based food, amount should not be your initial concern. The amount of water-based food that you eat is not the problem. Do you get it? One more time. The amount of water-based food that you eat is not the problem. For forty years I have been trying to get people to understand this. It has been maddening to me! So one more time. The amount of water-based food that you eat is not the problem. If you eat healthy foods consistently in whatever amount feels right and you don't resort to institutional dieting or some special formula with chemical shakes and bars, your body is going to change how it reacts in terms of cravings, needs, and overall social behavior. You will experience food situations where there may be no great options, and you may slip up. But it is important that you realize you are not on a time-based institutional diet. The dynamic you are engaging involves changing your overall food-related behavior incrementally.

Your food intake will begin to reflect your day. Whether you've had a sedentary day at the office or a physically demanding day working out or in the backyard, the healthy fuel will not create that craving for excess that was the result of your unhealthy intake. Your body will seek food amounts that are correct and balanced. This moderation in intake of good food in combination with increased activity induces a system cleansing that allows you to feel better now and to learn how to adjust and readjust your levels of good food intake and activity to your lifestyle. You learn to do this not by prescribing amounts of food but by eating water-based foods and engaging in fitness activity. Mindfulness of your body's progressive response to this cleansing will help you customize your food intake at a level adequate to the demands of your lifestyle. Setting the amount that you should eat is just not part of this process. It is rather a constant awareness of body and mind. The more you train the better you get.

Calories

What is a calorie? Should we care? How much should we care? What is it with this obsession about calories? It is something I have had to deal with since the beginning of New Life. From then until now, people have always asked me how many calories are in the food. The number of calories is not the focus. Let me play out two scenarios for you.

The first scenario is that you are on an evening out in New York City at a fine restaurant. At this restaurant, you enjoy a nice calamari appetizer, some wonderful bread, beef Wellington with a side of green beans dipped in oils, a rich buttered potato with cheese, some red wine, and maybe finish it off with some cognac and chocolate mousse for dessert. Now you've left the restaurant, and you're feeling satisfied. You walk your way home and reach into your coat pocket for your keys. There your fingers find a Godiva chocolate bar with almonds that you bought earlier. You examine it with interest, noticing it has about three hundred calories. Then you say, "Why not?" and you eat it.

In the second scenario, you are away on an island tour. Oh no! You've been left behind and are stranded. Days later they finally realize you are missing and come looking for you. The rescue team finds you, and the first thing they see is that you need food. The rescuer offers you a chocolate bar with almonds that also has three hundred calories.

Now the difference between these two scenarios comes down to the metabolism that occurs in each instance. Because of your sumptuous dinner, the first scenario includes an overabundance of fat and simple sugars or carbohydrates. Your body has nothing to do with these and dumps them in your pond merely to add to your girth. In the second scenario, your body needs the candy bar for energy. It's not the cleanest fuel, but it's used as fuel nonetheless and improves how you feel almost immediately.

These are two drastically varying scenarios, but you can see the way in which the number of calories—three hundred in these cases—is relative and not absolute in any objective way. A calorie is a unit of heat energy and perhaps even meaningless in terms of nurturing your pond. Forget about it! Letting go of counting calories and the focus on weight loss are the two biggest concepts to let go of to truly embrace *authentic wellness*. Again, what really matters is whether the food you are eating is water-based real food.

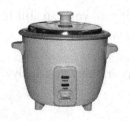

The Rice Maker

Growing up, our family would buy food that was inexpensive with very little nutritional value. For many families this is still true today. My best meal of the day came from the dollar that bought my school lunch. Had I known then what to do, I would have bought a rice maker. Not only is the rice cooker a low-cost item, but it's also convenient. You can just leave it cooking and do something else, maybe even exercise. Food can never be overcooked.

- Using the rice maker, add one and a half cups of brown rice and one-half cup of lentils with four cups of water. Then press the on button. Go for a walk, relax or get some chores done. Then forty minutes later you have a rice lentil dish to combine with canned kidney or black beans. With parmesan cheese, your chose of vegetables and favorite herbs and spices, this is a very nutritious meal that is inexpensive, tasty, and convenient. During the final fifteen minutes, you could place vegetables or leftover chicken to steam on the firm rice bed that has formed on the rice surface. You can use other options with the rice like canned tomatoes, or coconut milk in combination with the water base. This is nutritious food, convenient to prepare, has low cost, and will change your metabolism. Remember that in the beginning of this change, it doesn't matter how much real food you eat because real food will change your metabolism.

Decisions at Restaurants

Restaurants are by far the most common trap for would-be healthy eaters. Americans are accustomed to sugar, fat, and salt eating, and restaurants cater to that taste. If there's a nearby restaurant with good health food, that's great. If not, you can still find something to eat on a restaurant menu. I'll show you how.

First, here are some general tips that apply to all restaurants.

- Order à la carte. Full dinners usually add up to a lot of food, more than you need or even want. Try the hard test of leaving food on your plate when you feel full. Notice how it makes you feel.

- Watch out for soups. Clear soups usually are extremely high in salt. White creamy soups will be made with whole cream and perhaps with a canned base that is very fatty and high in salts. Restaurants, even fancy ones, use packaged food products called "ham base," "chicken base," and so on to flavor the stocks from which they make soups and sauces. The *base* contains fat, salt, sugar, and artificial flavorings. I call it "glop." I used this stuff when I was a cook. In restaurants I'm wary of soup.

- Limit fried foods and breaded foods. These will usually be cooked in a fryolator, and the oil is not changed very often, depending on the restaurant.

- Be careful about pastas. Many pasta sauces are made with a lot of fats and cream sauces with whole cream. They'll both be fat-dense.

- Ask for salad dressing on the side so that you may use as little as you want. Ask for oil and vinegar or lemon juice.

- Ask the server not to leave a bread basket at your table. It's very tempting when it's sitting right in front of you. If you do have it, try to limit butter or olive oil. Do not use margarine or other butter substitutes. The bread on the table will give you a chance to get in touch with your emotions about food. If I say, "Don't have the bread," notice how you feel about that. I was having lunch with an old friend I grew up with and had not seen in many years. He had no desire for the bread, but I wanted it so badly and noticed how it made me feel. I finally could not handle it and had some. He didn't. We have so many subjective feelings about food. To change, we should become aware of these feelings and change them at our own pace for the good of our pond.

- Ask your server what is in a dish or a sauce instead of guessing. You may find yourself with something you don't really want. Ask for the sauce on the side.

- Don't use wishful thinking. Just because you make your omelet with a small amount of butter doesn't mean the restaurant does.

- Order a couple of appetizers instead of a main course. Appetizers contain a smaller quantity of food, and some choices are fresher than entrées. However, most have lot of sugar, fat, and salt.

- Ask to have food prepared the way you want it. If fish is on the menu, ask them to broil it, but be sure to ask in advance.

- Try to get fruit for dessert. Often a menu will serve a fruit cup or melon as an appetizer but not list it as a dessert. If you ask for it as dessert, however, they will usually be happy to cooperate. If you wish and don't go out a lot, you can treat yourself to dessert.

- When the waiter says, "Would you like a side of french fries, coleslaw, or a fruit cup, notice how you react in your mind. You want the french fries, but you know the fruit cup is the water-based choice. But you want the french fries with the ketchup. Making the switch to the fruit cup is a significant emotional transformation. It can make you feel uncomfortable. After you try it a few times, you will get used to it. You may still want those french fries, but you are getting used to the fruit cup. You can also compromise and have the coleslaw. This is an example of getting in touch with the psychology of eating. You know what is best for your pond, but your habits are so mentally ingrained and you like the taste of the french fries. This is a major transformation. It might take a while. It might never happen, or it might only happen sometimes. Notice how many times during the day you have this same emotional conflict about food.

- Leaving food on your plate. Restaurants give you big portions, or you might be at an all-you-can-eat restaurant situation. Try to leave food on your plate when you are feeling full. Do you think you could eat only until you are full at an all-you-can-eat restaurant? For most that would be worse than torture. Can you handle not getting your money's worth? How much is your money's worth? Notice how you feel in these situations, and change will happen.

That's my basic bag of tricks. You may have some of you own, and no doubt, you'll develop more. In the meantime, I'd like to show you how I apply these tricks to a real menu.

A nice but not terribly expensive neighborhood restaurant provides our first menu. This is the sort of place you'd go for a business lunch or an informal dinner with friends. Start looking down this menu. For lunch, you might consider an omelet. If so, order it with spinach, onions, or mushrooms, not cheese or ratatouille (probably made with plenty of oil). If you're there for dinner, order fish and request it broiled without butter. The Poulette Supreme has bacon, cheese, and Bordelaise sauce (made from a traditional roux), all of which you're better off without. The sautéed calf's liver will be high in cholesterol (and the chemicals that have collected in the liver), but it's high in nutrients, so if you like it, order it. I'd suggest you do this only in a good restaurant where you know the liver is fresh, and I'd also recommend you have it without the bacon. The steak is better than the spareribs unless you really want it.

Regarding the appetizers, smoked trout, avocado vinaigrette (dressing on the side if possible), mussels (if fresh), and stuffed mushrooms are your best choices. The black bean soup sounds good, but it is probably made with the fatty stock base, which is a gamble I wouldn't take. The same goes for onion soup. Quiche is eggs, butter, and cream. Calamari fritti and fried wonton are fried food, and sparerib is pork—are not good choices.

Of the entrées, the deli sandwich (without pastrami), the vegetarian sandwich, the vegetable platter, mixed vegetable oriental, mussels marinara, and the club sandwich (on whole wheat bread) are the best. Some of these might have more cheese than you'd like. Remove it and leave it on your plate. The other entrées are either red meat or fried foods. Another thing about this menu is that many of the dishes are served with french fries. Ask to have a baked potato instead, or tell the waiter just to omit the french fries. If you don't mind being a bit annoying, you can ask for a side of vegetables.

Of the pastas, only the Capellini D'Angelo begins to fit the bill, but it's essentially egg noodles likely covered with an oil sauce. I'd pass up the pastas on this menu.

Three of the salads are fine—bean sprout, spinach, and chicken salad nicoise. Always ask for dressing on the side. Tabbouleh, if made the traditional way, will be very oily. Caesar salad has a fatty dressing that's extremely salty because of the anchovies. Feta cheese or Caponata salads are too cheesy, and the Mediterranean salad has red meat and cheese. Mussels with a vegetarian sandwich would be a great combo. If you really want some meat, ask them to put a few slices of turkey with it. The bean sprout salad would be good. Ask them to add some chicken or salmon, and you can pay the difference.

As for beverages, have decaf coffee, herbal tea, juice, seltzer, or sparkling cider.

Lunch only	Appetizers	Salads
Omelets	Black bean soup	Tabbouleh salad *Corn, bulgur wheat, cucumber and scallions in mint and lemon sauce.*
Plain	Onion soup	Bean sprout salad *Bean sprouts, watercress, scallions, mushrooms and water chestnuts with sesame dressing.*
Cheese (Swiss, cheddar, or gruyere)	Quiche du jour	Caesar salad
Ratatouille	Smoked trout	Spinach salad *Spinach, mushrooms, bacon and house dressing.*
Spinach	Avocado vinaigrette	Feta cheese salad

Onion	Calamari fritti	Caponata, tabbouleh and feta cheese salad
Mushroom	Mussels marinara	Whole smoked trout plate
Omelets served with fresh-cut french fries and salad.	Whole stuffed mushrooms	Chicken salad nicoise *Baked breast of chicken, artichoke hearts, zucchini, tomatoes, black olives, house dressing.*
Steak and eggs	Fried wonton	Mediterranean salad *Julienned salami, ham, cheese, onion, Tuscan peppers and tomatoes.*
Eggs francaise	Hacked spareribs	*Salads served with french bread and sweet butter.*
Eggs Benedict		
Eggs Florentine	**Entrées**	**Pasta**
Above entrées served with fresh-cut french fries.	Deli sandwich *Pastrami, melted cheese, grilled tomato and onion on whole grain bread.*	Capellini D'Angelo (angel hair pasta) *Ultra-fine imported egg noodles dressed with sundried tomatoes, lightly sautéed in garlic flavored olive oil.*
	Vegetarian sandwich *Melted cheese with bean sprouts, tomato and onion on whole grain bread.*	Fettuccini white *Egg noodles, heavy cream and aged parmesan cheese.*

Dinner only	House burger *Hamburger, with or without jalapeño peppers and melted cheese on toasted French Bread.*	Fettuccini red *Egg noodles in tomato and meat sauce.*
Fish du jour	Steak sandwich *Broiled sliced shell steak on toasted French bread with bordelaise or mustard and garlic sauce.*	Small order of fettuccini
Poulette supreme *Boneless breast of chicken stuffed with country bacon and gruyere cheese served with bordelaise sauce.*	*Above sandwiches served with fresh-cut French Fries and salad.*	Pasta del giorno
Sautéed calves liver *with bacon and onion.*	Vegetable platter *Stuffed mushrooms, ratatouille and vegetable du jour.*	
Broiled shell steak	Mixed vegetable oriental *Fresh vegetables sautéed with soy sauce, garlic and ginger with rice.*	
Steak au poivre *Shell steak with peppercorns cooked in a brandy and cream sauce.*	Mussels marinara *Mussels steamed in white wine, garlic and butter.*	

Above entrées served with salad, vegetable and potato or rice.	Calamari fritti	
Barbecue spareribs *With black bean salad and rice.*	Club sandwich *Turkey, bacon, lettuce and tomato on French bread.*	
	Hamburger solo	

Now let's try Chinese food at a popular neighborhood restaurant serving Szechuan cuisine. The first and most important rule about eating in a Chinese restaurant is to ask for food without monosodium glutamate (MSG). If more and more people request no MSG, eventually Chinese restaurants will stop using it. Many have. Another rule is to ask what things are. Some menus explain the dishes, but if you're unsure, ask. The servers are trained to answer, and it's the only way to know what you're getting.

From this menu, for a dinner for four, I would probably order the following: wonton or egg drop soup, cold noodles with sesame sauce, mixed vegetables, pineapple chicken or paradise chicken, dragon meets phoenix, or assorted seafood delight. (I'd ask about this one first.) These dishes look like the *purest* and seem to have the lightest sauces. I tend to avoid highly spiced foods, believing with the yogis that it's best to eat more *neutral* foods. That is only my choice, of course, and you can certainly eat spicy foods if you like them. But be sure you're getting spices and not oily sauces.

Other dishes among the appetizers I might choose are plain noodles Szechuan style, noodles Peking style, paper-wrapped chicken, any of the vegetarian choices, or any of the poultry except sweet and sour chicken or crispy fried duck. Of the specialties, I'd have prawns and scallop combination, sliced chicken with fermented rick sauce, empire special garden vegetables, or aromatic Chinese eggplant. Of the seafood, I'd have any except fried dishes or those with heavy sauces. The only way to tell about most of these dishes is to ask before you order. For instance, sliced prawns with snow peas may be fine. But if the server tells you it's in a white sauce, don't order it. White sauce will probably be made with corn starch, which is heavy and nutritionally empty. Lemon chicken may be all right, but it might also be breaded.

Skip fried rice or noodles. Ask for brown rice. However, white rice may be all they serve. Have fruit for dessert. Drink seltzer or club soda instead of sugared sodas.

Appetizers	**Golden chicken with five flavors** Diced chicken buttered with water chestnut powder and then deep fried and drained. Then sautéed with five flavor sauce (wine, sugar, soy sauce, hot pepper, oil and vinegar, no MSG).
Hot spicy Chinese cabbage	**Empire special duck** Sliced boneless duck breaded in snow pea, winter bamboo shoot, red bell pepper and water chestnut.
Fried or boiled dumpling (8)	**Dragon meets phoenix** Chunks of unshelled lobster, sliced chicken white meat, red bell pepper, baby corns and black mushroom in delicious light sauce.
Fried wonton (8)	**Unshelled lobster and beef** Chunks of unshelled lobster, sliced flank steak, broccoli, red bell pepper and straw mushrooms in garlic sauce.
Spare ribs (small to large)	**Crispy prawns Szechuan style** Crispy fried prawns showered with chef's special Szechuan sauce. Green broccoli on the side.
Egg roll (1)	**Scallops among black pearls** Sliced Scallops, straw mushrooms, baby corns and sliced ham sautéed with hot Hunan sauce.
Shrimp toast (4)	**Duet of scallop and beef** Delicious combination of scallop and sliced flank steak sautéed with scallion and water chestnut in oyster Kung-pao sauce.
Barbecued beef Szechuan style (2)	**Assorted seafood delight**

Pu pu platter (for 2)	**Wo bar trio** Sizzling wo-bar with prawns, scallops and sliced chicken with snow pea pods, carrot and water chestnut.
Cold bean curd with hot sesame oil	
Cold noodles with sesame sauce	**Seafood**
Plain noodles Szechuan style	Lobster Cantonese style
Noodles Peking style	Sautéed lobster Szechuan style
Paper wrapped chicken (4)	Hot braised lobster
Hacked chicken with multiflavor	Sliced prawns with snow peas
	Sliced prawns with garlic sauce
Soup	Prawns with barbecued sauce
Wonton soup	Prawns with chili sauce
Egg drop soup	Empires special shrimp
Hot and sour soup	Shrimp with lobster sauce
Bean curd with mushroom soup	Fried shrimp
Shredded pork with Szechuan pickled cabbage	Plain sautéed baby shrimp
	Sautéed baby shrimp with dried red pepper
Vegetarian Choices	Baby shrimp sautéed with green peas
Dried sautéed string beans	Baby shrimp with garlic sauce
Sautéed bamboo shoots and mushrooms	Sautéed shrimp with chili sauce
Mushrooms Szechuan style	Sautéed shrimp with bean curd
Mixed vegetables	Sweet and sour prawns
Eggplant with garlic sauce	Sautéed diced chicken and shrimp
Broccoli with garlic sauce	Shrimp with cashew nuts
Bean curd Szechuan style	Scallops with hot garlic sauce
Bean curd home style	Scallops sautéed

Bean curd with black bean sauce	Scallops with dried red pepper
	Sautéed scallops with chili sauce
Pork	sautéed scallops with black bean sauce
Moo shu pork (pancake)	Sweet and sour fish
Sliced pork doubly sautéed	Spicy crispy fried fish
Pork sautéed with broccoli	
Pork sautéed with scallions	**Beef and Lamb**
Sweet and dour pork	Beef with mushrooms and bamboo shoots
Shredded pork with Peking sauce	Beef sautéed with broccoli
Shredded pork with garlic sauce	Beef with snow seas
	Beef in orange flavor
Poultry	Beef with scallions
Ta-chien chicken	Beef with barbecue sauce
Chicken in orange flavor	Shredded beef with dried hot pepper
Sliced chicken with snow peas	Shredded beef with hot chili sauce
Moo go gai pan	Shredded beef with green pepper
Sliced chicken with garlic sauce	Shredded beef with garlic sauce
Diced chicken with dried red pepper	Shredded beef with Peking sauce
Diced chicken with bean sauce	Shredded beef with bean sauce
Sweet and sour chicken	Pepper steak
Diced chicken with cashew nuts	Sliced lam Hunan style
Showered chicken with ginger sauce	Sautéed lamb with scallions
Crispy fried duck (half)	
	Fried Rice
Specialties	Ten ingredients fried rice

Lamb with Szechuan ma la sauce Sliced lamb, broccoli, baby corns, and shredded bell pepper sautéed with Szechuan ma la sauce.	Fried rice with (shrimp, chicken, beef or pork)
Prawns and scallop combination A delicious array of sliced prawns and scallops, straw mushroom, snow pea pods and bell pepper sautéed with delicious hot sauce.	
Sliced chicken with fermented rice sauce Sliced tender chicken breast, woods ear mushroom snow pea pods and red bell peppers sautéed with fermented sweet rice sauce.	**Noodles**
Empire three delicates sautéed Sliced prawns, sliced chicken, sliced pork and scallion sautéed with bean sauce.	Ten ingredients lo mein
Pineapple chicken Sliced white meat, pineapple cubes, red bell pepper, woods ear mushrooms, broccoli and green peas in tasty light sauce.	Lo mein with (shrimp, chicken, beef, or pork)
Paradise chicken Sliced white meat chicken, red bell pepper, and watercress sautéed with hot Szechuan sauce.	Fried rice noodles

Empire special garden vegetables A splendid array of vegetables enhanced by a bed of lotus stem woods ear mushrooms, glutton of wheat, snow pea pods, broccoli and tomato in hot sauce.	
Aromatic Chinese eggplant Small Chinese eggplant sautéed with garlic, scallion and pepper in rich aromatic sauce (no MSG).	

Next, consider a somewhat fancier dinner restaurant with an Italian accent. Of the appetizers on this menu, the clams, shrimp cocktail (eat the sauce sparingly), mussels, and tomato juice are the best. Antipasto has red meat, cheese, and oil. Prosciutto is like ham made from pork legs. An old classic but not so healthy for modern times. The melon alone would be good. Clams casino are breaded. Soup is a gamble.

Of the entrées, avoid prime rib and veal francaise, The other veal dishes are all right, but you might ask them to go easy on the butter. Any of the seafood is okay, but you might ask that it be broiled. Don't order any of the Italian entrées. The veal, chicken, and eggplant parmigiana are breaded and have a rich cheese sauce. The pastas are all heavy and cheesy. With your entrée, you get a vegetable (fine), a baked potato (with cottage cheese or limited butter or sour cream), and salad (dressing on the side). Have fruit or nothing for dessert.

If I were eating here, my first choice would be to order appetizers instead of a main course. I would have a house salad to start asking for additional vegetable they might have. Then I'd have clams on the half shell and a shrimp cocktail. With them, I'd have a baked potato (with cottage cheese and pepper or a little butter). This would probably be plenty of food, the two appetizers equaling one entrée. I might have fruit for dessert. Maybe they could give me a piece of melon since they have it available.

My second choice would be to start with a salad and then have veal scaloppini, piccata or marsala, or one of the four suitable seafood dishes with a baked potato. (I'd also ask the chef to decrease the butter.) Again, I'd want fruit for dessert. Oh, what the heck. I would have dessert.

Appetizers	
Lg Antipasto	Sm antipasto
Clams on half shell	Clams casino
Shrimp cocktail	Mussels (in season)
Prosciutto and melon	Chilled tomato juice
Soup du jour	
Entreés	
Roast prime ribs of beef au jus *a hearty cut of prime beef with a baked potato*	
Veal saltimbocca sautéed veal with prosciutto ham-mozzarella cheese *in a white wine-butter and lemon sauce*	
Veal scaloppini *sautéed veal in mushrooms-white wine with red sauce*	
Veal piccata *sautéed veal in butter-lemon with white wine*	
Veal marsala *sautéed veal in butter-mushrooms and marsala wine*	
Veal Francoise *sautéed veal dipped in egg with a lemon butter and white wine sauce*	
Seafood scampi *flounder, shrimp & scallops broiled in white wine lemon, garlic, and butter sauce*	
Shrimp scampi *4 jumbo shrimp butterflied and broiled in white wine, lemon, and butter*	

Flounder Francoise *filet of flounder dipped in egg and sautéed with white wine, lemon, and butter*
Broiled flounder *filet of flounder broiled in a lemon and butter sauce*
Broiled scallops *broiled scallops in a butter sauce*
Veal parmigiana *breaded cutlet of veal baked with sauce and mozzarella cheese*
Chicken parmigiana *breaded boneless breast of chicken baked with sauce and mozzarella cheese*
Eggplant parmigiana *pan fried eggplant baked with sauce and mozzarella cheese*
Lasagna *stuffed with meat-ricotta cheese and baked with tomato sauce*
Baked manicotti *stuffed noodles with ricotta-mozzarella and baked with tomato sauce*
Fettuccine alfredo *wide noodles with a special basil and cheese sauce*

A natural foods restaurant will make it easier to find wholesome nutritious foods on this menu. Of the appetizers, hummus, skinny dip, and Japanese vegetable soup (a miso broth) are best. The magic mushrooms look good but might be oily. (Pesto sauce is made with a good deal of oil.) Guacamole is made with avocado, so enjoy! The nacho chips are fried. I would ask about the moose caboose. Depending on how the salmon mousse is made, this could be terrific. The Paprikash potatoes, however, are probably fried, and the sour cream is too high in fat.

All the salads are probably fine, except Athena's. That has cheese and will be too salty with olives and anchovies. At a natural food restaurant, I would expect the tabbouleh not to be too oily. The Middle East feast would be okay. Pesto sauce, as I said before, tends to be oily and fatty with cheese, nuts, butter, and oil, but on a large salad eaten as an entire meal, it may be okay. The garden house and garden party salads are perfect.

Any of the entrées would be fine too. The pumpkin platter with no sauce is the purest. The exotic curry with cashew sauce is the heaviest. But you'd really be all right with any of them. Avoid quiche (eggs, cheese, and cream). As for soup, in this restaurant it is probably not made with the glop, and so it will be fine. The thing to really watch out for in a health food restaurant is too much cheese. Ask the kitchen to use less cheese or remove it (if it's layered on top) when your order arrives. Notice the sides that are offered. In this case the steamed vegetables, brown rice, beans, and bread would all be good choices.

Drink any juices, teas, or decaf coffee. The smoothies would be fine and very nutritious.

Appetizers—plate pleasers	
Tabbouleh	Cracked wheat, diced vegetables and lemon juice.
Heavenly hummus	A creamy treat of chick peas, tahini and lemon served with pita wedges and a warning: may be habit forming.
Magic mushrooms	Fresh pesto stuffed caps sprinkled with parmesan and broiled to perfection.
Great guacamole	A tangy avocado-herb blend surrounded by nacho chips.
Nutty noodles	Cold Soba noodles with creamy ginger-peanut sauce garnished with cucumber and scallion.
The skinny dip	Crunchy crudité served with a precious pot of our special sauce.
Paprikash potatoes	Topped with sour cream and scallion.

Savory soups
Japanese vegetable
Daily variety

Garden path	
Athena's salad	Fresh feta, crisp cucumber, olives, onion, tomato and anchovies atop romaine lettuce.
Middle east feast	Creamy hummus and tabbouleh garnished with olives and pita atop romaine lettuce.
Pasta potpourri	Tasty tortellini tossed with assorted vegetables and our special pesto sauce served cold.
Garden house	A bed of romaine and cabbage with julienne carrots, cucumber, tomato and a finishing touch of scallion and chick peas.
Garden party	A larger house embellished with mushroom, pepper and broccoli. Add tuna, guacamole, sprouts or "the works" our chefs' special with guacamole, tabbouleh, tuna and cheese.

Ocean potions (served with garden house salad)	
Pumpkin patch catch	Fresh filet of the day, broiled and served with paprikash potatoes or rice and steamed vegetables.
Bonsai bluefish	Sliced fish and vegetables sautéed in a garlic and lemon sauce over rice.
Bluefish sesame	Fresh filet rolled in sesame seeds, broiled, served with rice and steamed vegetables.
Filled salmon	Fresh filed broiled in a light dill sauce with paprikash potatoes or rice and steamed vegetables.
Flower of the seas	Filets rolled around broccoli and stuffed with tomato, parsley and minced scallion with rice.

Great plates for the pampered palate (served with our garden house salad)	
Oriental express	Snow peas, mushroom, Chinese cabbage, onion and bean curd sautéed and covered with ginger-peanut sauce served on noodles.

Exotic curry	Seasonal vegetables and chick peas in creamy cashew sauce over brown rice, topped with chopped apricots and currants with cucumber raita, chutney and crispy lentil bread.
Pasta primavera	Seasonal vegetables, olives, onion and tomatoes sautéed and tossed with fettuccini noodles in a garlic herb sauce, topped with parmesan.
Tasty tostada	Beans, cheese and vegetables sitting on a corn tortilla covered with tomato salsa and a dab of guacamole.
Wok way	Assorted vegetables sautéed in ginger-tamari herb sauce with a meat-like soy protein over brown rice.
Garden platter	Steamed seasonal vegetables over brown rice with melted cheese or creamy ginger peanut sauce sprinkled with sesame seeds and scallion.
Earth burger	A nutritious meat like protein patty broiled served with steamed vegetables and brown rice with your choice of creamy ginger peanut sauce or tomato sauce and cheese.
Pumpkin platter	Assorted steamed vegetables, brown rice our bean of the day and salad with tahini dressing.
Quiche and garden house salad	
Savory soup and a garden house salad	
Side steps	Steamed vegetables Brown rice Beans Bread Sauces

At a roadside restaurant, a diner, a chain such as Friendly's, TGI Fridays, Denny's, a fast-food place (McDonalds, Taco Bell, etc.), or a pizza joint, you'll have a much harder time. If they have a salad bar, you're safe, but avoid the extras—the bacon bits, cheeses, macaroni salad, pudding, and others—and stick with a simple dressing. If there's no salad bar, perhaps you can have a fruit and cottage cheese salad (decline the Jell-O) or a tuna or chicken sandwich on whole wheat bread.

It is amazing to me how many pizza options you have. I've progressed from the days I ate package pizza as a teenager to then enjoying the classic New York City slice to creating a whole wheat pita pizza at New Life. We see a million-dollar advertisement on the Super Bowl with the pizza that costs less the ten dollars. The ingredients must be so cheap. Learn which pizza fits into your healthy transformation.

At this point, it may seem like an awful lot of work to analyze every menu you're handed. With a little practice though, it becomes second nature. It takes me a minute or less to scan a menu and pick out the desirable items. In fact, looking at a menu critically makes it easier to decide what to order because so many things are usually out of the question. Give it a try and see if you aren't happier about eating out. You won't be stuffed and bloated, and therefore, you won't be annoyed with yourself. It will be good for your girth circumference.

Most of the time, it is possible to eat well even when you're eating out. But again, don't be discouraged if you can't always do it. If you're having lunch with a person who likes fried mozzarella sticks with fried fish and french fries and who also happens to be a potential major client, you may not want him or her to question your sanity when you order two appetizers. In that case, eat whatever seems most sensible, perhaps salad and fish. If you're taken out to a surprise birthday dinner where they present you with a luscious rich chocolate cake made and decorated by your friends, it would be rude to not eat a piece. Your pond is very resilient; it will recover. At the next meal or the next day, you can find other ways to integrate more water-based food using the information and strategies that you have learned.

The "Only One Cookie" Situation

My favorite example to illustrate our relationship with food is based on two groups of people. This can be understood by buying a box of your favorite cookies. Mine are the ones with chocolate chips and walnuts. They do have a bit of nutrients because of the nuts. Store them in the cupboard. Group one can have two cookies with some tea and then put the cookies back in the cupboard and forget about them. Most of my guests at New Life and I make up the second group. This is one of the reasons I am in business. This group will not just have two cookies but will eat the whole box whether they are hungry or not. Which are you?

We have learned to not have the cookies in the house. If you want to be a thin person, you do what thin people do. You eat when you're hungry. But as I said, we don't eat mostly when we are hungry. We don't even know what real hunger is. We live in a culture with a lot of food and even more nonfood. In certain environments, we can't really control ourselves in terms of that feeling, and we don't know whether we are hungry or not. So why can't you just say no to the cookies? You may feel you need discipline, but we have not really defined discipline. You may now realize that changing eating habits is multidimensional and subjective.

What I find interesting is that we kind of laugh about this issue and never really delve into why this is so. I think we should spend some time and energy on examining this mental state. But as I said, this transformation is an individual process. The government or a research group will probably not help.

I have changed over decades of personal growth to avoid institutional dieting, and I have learned the psychology and emotions related to my own personal transformation. I am much better at not having the cookies when they are in the cupboard. I still feel the desire throughout my body, but I react to it less and less.

I have made this transformation by examining and working through the psychology and emotions of this desire to eat all the cookies. Because of this dysfunction, I spent a lot of time examining this. Someone who came from a less unsettled childhood environment might not feel the need to explore this area as much as I needed to, but they still might need to change to become a more water-based person.

When you are willing to change by putting real food into your body, you will change your body chemistry, which will change the mind and your emotional and psychological relationship with food. You will begin to feel real hunger, and you will not have to finish everything on your plate or buy the candy bars and other nonfoods just because you feel emotional drawn to them. You won't feel mad at yourself about situations where you eat food that you know is not good for you, and you will feel this change as a process. With real food in your body, the emotions will slowly dissolve.

The other thing to remain cognizant of as we move forward is how very subjective, personal, and individual the mental and emotional constructs that characterize and define your relationship with food. These are very unique to you. Let's delve a bit deeper now to touch on the psychology of our relationship with food. The importance of doing so will set a new foundation for behavioral changes that conform to the discovery of your own path to *authentic wellness*.

CHAPTER 4

The Psychology

Abundance Out of Control

Let's do a thought experiment about the abundance of food available to us, though most of it is without nutritional value. Let's consider the possible places, big and small, that sell food in our town or city. These food sources include but may not be limited to big-box stores, department stores, supermarkets, pharmacies, convenience stores, health food stores, fine dining and other restaurants, diners, farmer's markets, lunch counters, food trucks, greasy spoons, truck stops, school lunch programs, hospitals, movie theaters, vending machines, Girl Scout cookies and other fundraisers, and any produce gardens. Let's place all the food in the local park and do a computer analysis of the nutrition available in all this food in relation to its impact on the population of the town or city. Consumption of this food places the population on a track to obesity and major degenerative diseases. This eating pattern is not sustainable both because of the personal health effects and because of the increasing costs to our health care system.

The change in our food supply over the last sixty-seven years has had a dramatic effect on our health. This change occurred after food manufacturers determined that the cheapest foods to make were those that contained large amounts of salt, fat, and sugar and that this increased appeal to consumers. The overuse of salt is a major factor in high blood pressure. The overuse of fat is a major factor in heart disease and stroke. The overuse of sugar is a major factor in diabetes. The effect of this overuse is an epidemic of degenerative disease that research has shown could be significantly decreased with changes in the foods we eat and a more active lifestyle.

Emotional Eating

Beyond the fundamentals, our discussion so far has encompassed the education, what real food is, how to obtain it, and the balance to consider for your fitness efforts, and the sociology, those behaviors and interactions that influence the decisions about food that you make in your ongoing life. The path to *authentic wellness* is multidimensional. Our discussion will now explore the psychology, the mental and emotional forces connected with food and eating. This extremely subjective (meaning personal and individual) nature of mental and emotional forces is what makes recognizing and changing food relationships and behaviors so difficult.

Simply understood, emotional eating is eating when you are not hungry. The abundance of food, the choices we have, and its availability mean that we are not familiar with hunger. As a result, we can eat for many reasons beyond hunger and nutritional needs. This is complicated further because most of the food choices available to us are unhealthy. We do like to eat. To make the change to a healthy eating lifestyle, we now will examine the complexities of overeating and the psychological dynamics involved in making that transition.

After graduate school I moved back to New York to set up a nutritional coaching practice. I knew many people in the metropolitan area who had been and continued to be New Life guests. Although I was not yet a certified therapist, I was qualified to offer nutritional coaching. This enabled me to apply my graduate studies to the people who wanted help with their food-related behavior patterns. In helping people to examine the mind-set underlying their food-related behavior, they would obtain insight conducive to choices about those behaviors. For me, the opportunity to examine the mind-set of food-related behaviors kept with my own life struggle with food issues. That struggle was mine too, and it rendered my wish to help others.

Additionally, my counseling experiences offered another window into the food and fitness perspectives that New Life continued to disclose to me. My practice provided a beacon to focus on mind-centered food behavior, and New Life provided a laboratory for the nutrition and fitness observations relevant to wellness. Together, my counseling practice and New Life combined to strengthen my abilities to understand and articulate the internal and the human dynamics that constituted the mind-body connection. The activation of the mind-body connection through the daily practice of a lifestyle of nutrition and fitness would help in the healing process and lead to *authentic wellness*.

My nutritional counseling consisted of ten sessions that guided the individual in examining the psychological, educational, and sociological elements that comprised the person's food-related behavior and environment. Our discussions permitted these individuals to identify foods they liked but were not healthy. Among those, we discussed which ones they chose to abandon and which they chose to keep. As the sessions progressed, they made choices about what would and would not remain in their food choices. The act of *choosing* rather than being restricted followed by a success in implementing their personal strategy made the individuals less fearful and more confident about their food-related behavior.

These individuals came to see that the personal success achieved in this food implementation had nothing to do with dieting and could not be standardized. The nutritional guidance in our discussion of the foods to continue was based on the premise that as the body was mostly water, foods rich in water should govern selection of foods to keep or eliminate. I also offered practical advice like label reading to identify ingredients to avoid, establishing a healthy food environment at home, and navigating the food behavior risks of social and business scenarios.

A Deeper Understanding

The psychological dynamics of the sessions fascinated me. Almost like clockwork, by the third session, individuals had encounter food-related issues based in childhood. The fact that childhood was the stage at which food-related issues originated was certainly not a novel discovery for me. However, an individual's surfacing and articulation of these cognitions developed from therapy offered the person the opportunity (from the vantage point of an adult frame of mind) to confront the anxieties he or she had harbored since childhood.

Once the individual could consider and articulate childhood food emotions from an adult perspective, with therapeutic guidance, the irrational behaviors could be understood and reformed over time. With the therapist's presence and support through an inevitable wave of discomfort, the individual could chip away at the old behaviors that had little to do with their present life situation. Letting go of these patterns is deeply rooted in body and mind. They would then feel more comfortable to select new food behavior patterns that contributed to the individual's immediate and future well-being.

The bonus to the individual in changing food-related behavior patterns was that these changes also resulted in changes in body metabolism. This was simply because the individual began to stop eating at least some of the foods that were unhealthy. The metabolic change was gradual and apparent only in retrospect over the course of the typical ten-week therapeutic period.

Self-Discipline and Personal Responsibility

Growth and personal transformation are about self-discipline. "Just do it!" or "Just say no!" are ways to change. But these are imperatives, commands that can be based on harshness and require stark self-control. Approaches to change that are rushed or prevent us from learning about ourselves as we experience change are not effective. Better are approaches to change that are based on practice of the activity and awareness of the thoughts and feelings being experienced as gradual improvement occurs. Practice might not take us all the way to perfection, but it will make us better progressively.

This route to change would be *authentic*. Rather than directed or imposed from sources outside of ourselves, authentic change is change for which we are our own source. It originates from within us. We are its authors. We authorize it. Authentic change is the foundation out of which the path to *authentic wellness* is crafted.

The enhancement of self-discipline and personal responsibility in our relationship with food involves emotional and psychological dimensions. The first of these is to accept that diets do not work. We should recognize that our relationship to food is unique because like drinking water, breathing, and sleeping, we must eat. Unlike addictions for which there are successful programs to keep people "clean" or "on the wagon," there are no equivalent programs for food that have proven successful in the long term.

Change in eating habits requires a change in the emotional and psychological patterns deeply etched into our mental construct from the time of our earliest eating experiences. These habits are so deeply ingrained that they act as negative filters in the subconscious mind to prevent change. The individual may not be aware of the filters. The individual may deny the filters. The individual may be aware of the filters and choose not to change. The individual may be aware of the filters and attempt to transform them. Because food is so much a part of our lives and the related feelings are so deeply seated in our minds, eating habits are the hardest of habits to change. It can be argued that our relationship to food goes deeper than addiction.

Dieting is a linear, mechanistic, authoritarian approach to change as opposed to the holistic dimensional approach I have recommended here. Attention to the deeply rooted psychological patterns characterizes a nonlinear approach. I did an extremely beneficial workshop at the Esalen Institute in Big Sur, California, during the mid-1980s, participating in a powerful therapeutic experience. Back then I began to understand that changing emotional patterns was a process that occurred on many levels over time. Gradual change in emotional patterns releases the past pain bound up in these emotions. The emotional release enables the body to divest itself of anxiety and enhances the opportunity for the mental filters that govern eating behaviors so that we can begin to dissipate and reform our behavior.

As this change progresses, the individual begins to make eating decisions less from anger, fear, lack of love, or other negative emotions. Instead eating decisions become more rooted in the actual sensation of hunger. The mind-body connection strengthens, and new pathways for change are established. The individual becomes different as the new pathways are integrated into his or her behavior. The self-discipline and personal responsibility required to change eating habits are made possible by this integrative dynamic.

Weight and Other Measures

When I first started New Life, I was always weighing and measuring people. I thought it was silly; however, it was a societal expectation of the times, and it was meaningful to people who were sincere in seeking change. This caused me to develop some strong feelings about scales and charts that recommend how much you should weigh. I think the best use for a scale is to see how much the package you are trying to send UPS weighs.

I have some other suggestions to evaluate your progress. Men may want to assess themselves by their pant size or the notches used in their belt. Women may want to measure themselves by fitting on articles of clothing that they haven't worn in a while. Try looking in the mirror without feeling scared and evaluating your girth circumference. How is your blood pressure, your usage of medication and antacid pills, and your overall bowl movement? These are significant indicators of the overall wellness of your pond.

The qualitative value of your energy is the most important indicator to understand. The quality of your life is determined by the extent of your energy to do the things that you want to do. There is no doubt that by eating water-based foods, whole proteins, and whole grains, you are giving yourself more natural energy and improving daily well-being and overall health.

In contrast to standing on a scale and dwelling on a number, it would be better to look at the bodies of those who populate the photos from before the 1950s when most foods were natural and water-based. Then examine photos of yourself or others from 1950 to the present. You can easily understand the changes formed in people's bodies by the shift toward processed foods. Since that time, this shift of historic proportion has characterized our culture.

CHAPTER 5

The Practicalities

Jekyll and Hyde and the Pig-Out

You work nine to five. You have a long commute. You travel a lot. Or maybe you are retired. One size cannot fit all. There are so many different schedules that we need a completely subjective, personal, individual, long-term approach to dealing with the epidemic of unhealthy eating.

It is 9:00 p.m., and you are hungry. In the kitchen there are all manner of possibilities—leftover cake, soda, bread, cookies, baloney, ice cream, frozen cheese cake, and more. Ideally, it would be best to not have any of this around. You know you shouldn't eat any of it. But it doesn't matter. You are out of control. In this state of mind, nothing you know intellectually is of consequence. You are in what I call the "Dr. Jekyll and Mr. Hyde syndrome." Only satisfying the craving matters, and you will turn into a lesser version of yourself in the quest for satisfaction. Carrots and celery will not cut it. This places you in the "pig-out mode." You eat … a lot. Later you may not feel so good about it emotionally or physically.

It's not the eating that's problematic. You should eat a lot if you want to. The point is *what* you are eating, not *that* you are eating. Choose healthy alternatives and nutritious substitutes such as ak-mak, pita bread, apple butter, tahini, 100 percent peanut butter, multigrain wraps, low-fat cheeses, yogurt, and fruit. The healthy alternatives are where to start when you pig out. If you start with these alternatives, food with real nutrition, your metabolism and body chemistry will change. You will not crave the unhealthy processed foods as much.

The food companies have helped you become addicted to the sugar, salt, and fat of unhealthy processed food. Load up the refrigerator and cupboard with healthy water based food—a lot of it. Don't be afraid to eat a lot of it, especially at the beginning. In the short term, you will be moving yourself in a new and healthy direction. In the long term, while you are improving your well-being, you will also be changing your pond and moving the food companies in a new and healthy direction.

If you must go to business lunches and cocktail parties during the week, try to cook healthy foods on the weekends. If you eat well during the week, maybe splurge on fine dining or a hot dog at a ball game. Whatever you do, try to eat with awareness. Don't feel guilty or say you have been bad. If you've had a hard day and you go home and eat a quart of ice cream and a box of cookies, don't panic. The next morning, eat a good breakfast and water-based food with many of the foods that have been recommended. This will even out your blood sugar level. If you've drank a bit too much or eaten a lot of peanuts or chips, you may feel slightly ill and not be hungry in the morning. But when you do begin to feel hungry, eat water-based foods. They'll go to work right away, give your body nutrients, and start to counteract the pollution in your body.

Holidays are often a problem, but the solution is the same. Eat water-based foods the next day. In many families, holiday dinners are sacrosanct. Still, if possible, try changing something. Have turkey instead of ham at Christmas. Switch to whole wheat bread. Cut down on the sugar and fat in fruit pies.

When you eat at a friend's house, you can't usually do much about what's being served. If you offer to bring a vegetable dish or a dessert, however, you'll be controlling at least that aspect of the meal and maybe introduce your friends to something new. But remember that a friend puts love and good energy in the preparation of that meal, and it won't hurt you. The psychological benefits of a meal shared with friends may outweigh the nutritional defects.

Sometimes you find yourself staying with friends or relatives for a week or more. You can't really say, "Yuck, this food is terrible. You eat all wrong here. I'm going to restock your kitchen." Aside from offering to prepare a meal or two, you can't do much except try to make the best choices you can. Make up for it when you get home. Another thing to remember is that even if you eat well every time you have control of your meals, you will still have plenty of opportunity to eat ice cream or chocolate eclairs because there will always be times when you're not in control—dinners out, parties, and business meals. It's about changing toward more water-based food.

The skill of making healthier food choices is vital in changing eating habits. It is also important to distinguish making healthier food choices from institutional dieting. A transformation customized by you for your own life situation and tastes is *not* dieting. Your food choices can, for example, be made on the extent to which your preferences favor or disfavor sugar, salt, and fat. Identifying those personal inclinations will contribute to your ability to change your eating habits. The next section of label reading will help in this transition.

Liquid Sugar Problem

For many years there has been a soda epidemic. It has circled the globe. Instead of addressing the epidemic, we have ignored the situation, and it has morphed into a more complex drink epidemic. Significant changes can occur to your body just by removing liquid sugar. Ultimately, the only liquid your body needs as fuel is water. It is the best source of pure hydration whether you're sitting in the office or out on a walk. Anything outside of water has been pushed into our lives by the global marketing culture, a manifestation of the wealth and sophistication of the food-industrial complex. Now this isn't to say that liquids can't carry healthy nutrients. As I said, teas, juices, and even vitamin C packets can be a nice change for your taste buds and supply overall benefit to your body, but water is all we need. In the following section includes examples of a variety of popular drinks available commercially.

Soda #1: Carbonated water, high fructose corn syrup, caramel color, phosphoric acid, natural flavors, caffeine.

Soda has been a leading factor in this negative paradigm shift in our nonfood lifestyle choices. It should be avoided as much as possible. It really is that simple. Sugar is sugar is sugar, and soda has lots of sugar that is not good for your pond.

Diet Soda #1: Carbonated water, caramel color, aspartame, phosphoric acid, potassium benzoate (to protect taste), natural flavors, citric acid, caffeine.

I remember when diet soda came on the scene. It was a miracle. A tasty drink with no calories. Marketing genius. From what I have learned, I would say that diet soda is like drinking a can of chemicals. Not sure what could be worse for your body and mind. There is a great deal of empirical data out there that also suggests diet soda is equally as unhealthy as real soda if not worse.

Sugar-Free Energy Drink #1: Carbonated water, citric acid, taurine, sodium citrate, magnesium carbonate, caffeine, glucuronolactone, acesulfame K, aspartame, inositol, niacinamide, calcium pantothenate, pyridoxine HCL, vitamin B12, xanthan gum, natural and artificial flavors, colors.

Energy drinks have skyrocketed in sales over recent years. This one is sugar-free, leaving out the leading ingredients, sucrose and glucose, that most have. The ingredients list is still left with an insane number of additives and unhealthful chemical compounds to load your body with. It's the ultimate drink used to create body highs that are impossible to maintain naturally. These swings can cause unhealthy changes to the body. So too, the caffeine dosages present can dehydrate your body.

Sports Drink #1: Water, sucrose, dextrose, citric acid, salt, sodium citrate, natural flavor, monopotassium phosphate, gum arabic, yellow 6, glycerol ester of rosin.

Sports drinks have a place. If you are competing at a high level, they will make your body more efficient for longer. That is the only place. You should not consume them as normal drinks. They contain dyes and additives that are unneeded but boost flavor and marketability. If you drink them when you are inactive, you are loading your pond with fuel that has nothing to do but become fat. Some sports drinks only recently removed brominated vegetable oil because of customer concern. It was first patented as a flame retardant. It helps hold together particles so that the ingredients don't separate. It is banned throughout Europe and Japan because it causes a whole array of bad side effects when ingested in high doses. It's worth checking to see if your drink contains this chemical.

Orange Juice #1: 100 percent pure pasteurized orange juice, calcium hydroxide, malic acid, citric acid, vitamin D3.

If you do want a sweet liquid, stick to juices. Watch out for added flavors and sugars. Plain 100 percent juice containing just juice does exist. Juices are at least based on natural sugars and real foods. Drinking too much juice when you are inactive can add to your girth. Have an orange or watermelon instead.

Seltzer #1: Carbonated water, natural flavors.

If bubbly is what you wanted, then this is the ideal substitute. If you feel this is bland, try half seltzer and half orange juice, apple cider, or grapefruit juice. You don't need to add sugar. This is a truly healthy alternative.

Teas, Coffee, Carrot Juice, Juicing

All in this section are true authentic options. I take that back. Not the Southern favorite. Sweet tea doesn't make the team. But herbal and regular teas do. Coffee is an American staple, even with a couple of teaspoons of sugar. It's best to go with milk over cream. Be careful to avoid the highs and lows caused by overuse. Before I started New Life, I worked with a group of doctors doing cardio stress tests. They told me how they had seen the effects of half-and-half and other creams on your blood, which is soon overcome with fat coursing through your body. The less fat, the better. Juicing is good but messy. Sometimes you can find bottled carrot juice. Cherry juice is worth it, but cherries are better.

Examples of how to read labels

The information listed on the box has very little value in understand what is in the product. It is the ingredient labeling that informs you what you are buying. Here are a few examples to better understand label reading.

Cereal #1: Milled corn, sugar, contains 2 percent of less of malt flour, salt, BHT for freshness.

You may like it when your milk tastes like sugar, but your body doesn't. The problem with most cereals is that they are loaded with sugar. This is your basic grain cereal coated with sugar. This is on par with dessert comparisons we will make later. At some point, marketing and a shift in the foods we bought led us to a place where we eat dessert for breakfast.

Cereal #2: Sugar, corn flour blend (whole grain yellow corn flour, degeminated yellow corn flour), wheat flour, whole grain oat flour, oat fiber, modified food starch, soluble corn fiber, contains 2 percent or less of hydrogenated vegetable oil (coconut, soybean and/or cottonseed), salt, natural flavor, red 40, tumeric extract color, yellow 6, blue 1, annatto extract color, BHT for freshness.

This is a classic case of dessert for breakfast. This cereal leads off with sugar. It contains all the dyes that are unusable materials within your body. Starting your day with a cereal like this for breakfast is hard to come back from. It creates a sugar rush, and you will inevitably crash. This is the repetitive process we are trying to avoid.

Cereal #3: Whole grain wheat flour, malted barley flour, isolated soy protein, salt, whole grain barley flour, malt extract, dried yeast. Vitamins and minerals: Reduced iron, niacinamide, zinc oxide (source of zinc), vitamin B6, vitamin A palmitate, riboflavin (vitamin B2), thiamin mononitrate (vitamin B1), folic acid, vitamin B12, Vitamin D.

This cereal, on the other hand, is 100 percent whole grain and consists of no sugar or unnecessary additives. This is a smarter way to start your day. It's high in fiber and has real fuel for your body to use, leading to less highs and lows that are caused by those other cereals.. Add banana, blueberries, or raspberries for added flavor. The purest box of cereal is spoon size shredded. Nothing but real wheat.

Bread #1: Whole wheat flour, water, bulgur wheat, sugar, wheat gluten, honey, soybean oil, yeast, whole wheat, salt, preservatives (calcium propionate, sorbic acid), monoglycerides, grain vinegar, datem, calcium sulfate, soy lecithin, natural flavors.

Here is a bread listed as 100 percent whole grain, a hundred calories per serving, and 12 percent of your daily fiber. These attributes are well-marketed positives, but when we look at the ingredients, we find that one of the top ingredients is sugar. This is an ongoing problem we face. Here is another food facet of our lives that is being infused with sugar. Now we compare this to the bread we use at New Life.

Bread #2: Sprouted organic whole wheat berries, filtered water, wheat gluten, honey, unsulphured molasses, cultured wheat, organic cracked wheat, organic cornmeal, organic millet, sea salt, fresh yeast, organic rye, organic sunflower seeds, organic oats, organic flax seeds, sunflower lecithin.

This is a real food ingredient label. No added ingredients are refined or chemicals. It really doesn't matter if the ingredients are organic. It matters that they are real food. Every ingredient in this product fits into authentic wellness. As you can see with the second bread, there is no unnecessary sugar. It derives its desired sweetness from natural honey alone. The second bread is also free of any long words that we would need to look up to understand. It is real food, the kind your body will appreciate.

Mac and Cheese #1: Enriched macaroni product (wheat flour, niacin, ferrous sulfate(iron), thiamin mononitrate (vitamin B1), riboflavin (vitamin B2), folic acid) cheese sauce mix (whey, milkfat, milk protein concentrate, salt, sodium tripolyphosphate, contains less than 2 percent of citric acid, lactic acid, sodium phosphate, calcium phosphate, yellow 5, yellow 6, cheese culture, enzymes).

Mac and cheese from a box doesn't have to be unhealthy. The previous example is though. Stepping away from the complicated words and additives, there is very little reason that we need dyes in macaroni and cheese. The color of the product is consistent as is, and we don't need to ingest a yellow dye 5 and 6.

Mac and Cheese #2: Macaroni (organic whole durum flour, filtered water), low fat milk, filtered water, reduced fat cheddar cheese (pasteurized milk, culture, salt, enzymes [without animal enzymes or rennet]), organic cornstarch, sea salt, mustard powder, organic annatto, spices.

This second macaroni and cheese removes the dye and additives and sticks to words you can understand. This is the real food that is good for your pond.

Pot Pies #1: Filling: Turkey broth (water, turkey flavor(turkey broth, salt, turkey fat, turkey meat, flavor)), turkey(turkey breast, water, isolated soy protein product(isolated soy protein, modified potato starch, corn starch, carrageenan, soy lecithin), dextrose, salt, seasoning(spice extractives, polysorbate 80, flavor)), carrots, peas, celery, modified corn starch, onions, contains 2 percent or less of soybean oil, salt, nonfat dry milk, cream, chicken broth powder (maltodextrin, chicken broth, salt, flavors), sugar, methylcellulose, flavoring, dried onions, xanthan gum, guar gum, extractives of turmeric. Crust: Enriched wheat flour(wheat flour, niacin, reduced iron, thiamine mononitrate, riboflavin, folic acid), interesterified soybean oil, water, salt, modified whey, caramel color.

This product is high in sodium, saturated fat, trans fats, and added sugars. What is methylcellulose and interesterfied soybean oil? Why is it in a turkey pot pie? Part of authentic wellness in learning to avoid these kind of ingredients and others like them.

Amy's Pot Pies—Pot Pies #2: Whole wheat flour, filtered water, butter, potatoes, carrots, tofu (filtered water, organic soybeans, magnesium chloride), onions, peas, sweet rice flour, tamari, water, soybeans, alcohol (to preserve freshness), salt, rice flour, sea salt, honey, spices, black pepper, yeast extract, turmeric.

This has real ingredients. These are the kinds of ingredients you are looking for. The healthy foodfreezer section of the grocery store contains many real food products. When it comes to premade foods though, the freezer section contains an abundance of products with unnatural additives and preservatives that are not needed in your body's pond. With close examination you can find products that have real ingredients. It is worth the time and energy.

Pizza #1: Enriched wheat flour (wheat flour, niacin, reduced iron, thiamin mononitrate, riboflavin, folic acid), water, fontina cheese (milk, cheese culture, salt, enzymes), low-moisture part-skim mozzarella cheese (part-skim milk, cheese culture, salt, enzymes), tomato paste, extra virgin olive oil, parmesan and pecorino Romano cheese blend (parmesan cheese(part-skim cow's milk, cheese cultures, salt, enzymes), pecorino Romano cheese (sheep milk, cheese cultures, salt, enzymes), salt, 2 percent or less of salt, sugar, herb blend (basil, oregano, thyme), yeast, malted barley flour, spice blend (salt, sugar, spices), garlic puree (garlic, vinegar), spice.

This has enriched wheat flour with lot of sugar, fat and salt. This food is doing you very little favors. It overloads your body with items you don't need. If you do have this kind of pizza try to supplement it with something healthy like a salad.

Amy's Pizza #2 (4 Cheese): Organic wheat flour with organic wheat germ and organic wheat bran, filtered water, organic tomato puree, mozzarella and parmesan cheeses (pasteurized part-skim milk, culture, salt, enzymes [without animal enzymes or rennet]), organic extra virgin olive oil, organic provolone cheese (organic pasteurized whole milk, culture, salt, enzymes [without animal enzymes or rennet]), organic honey, sea salt, expeller pressed high oleic safflower and/or sunflower oil, organic garlic, organic basil, organic red wine vinegar, pure organic cane sugar, spices, yeast.

This is what you are looking for. Again, it's not because of the organic foods but because the real ingredients have a healthy effect on your pond.

Dessert #1 (Oatmeal Raisin Cookie): Gluten-free oats, raisins, brown sugar, palm oil shortening, gluten-free flour (brown rice flour, potato starch, tapioca flavors), cane sugar, water, fructose, golden flaxseed, brown rice syrup, grape juice, rice dextrin, vanilla extract, baking soda, xantham gum, sea salt, sunflower lecithin, cinnamon.

A box of oatmeal raisin cookies is advertised as gluten-free and vegan. It also uses a good portion of the front of its box to exclaim that it's free of the top eight allergens (dairy, peanuts, eggs, tree nuts, wheat, fish, soy, and shellfish). On one side of the box, the brand explains its natural flavors—so much so that you might think it was a health food. Companies like to use healthy words and phrases, though the ingredients are not healthy for your pond. Words like gluten-free, vegan, allergens, and natural are used to manipulate healthy claims. This cookie may be a good allergen-free option for many with serious allergies. You might be allergic to wheat, but brown sugar, cane sugar, and fructose are all refined sugars. So too, palm oil is used in cosmetics, cleaning products, and a lot of unhealthy foods. Palm oil is right up there with my favorite nonfood oil, cottonseed oil.

Dessert #2 (Chocolate Cake): Filtered water, organic cane sugar, organic gluten-free flour (organic whole grain brown rice flour, organic rice flour, organic sorghum flour, organic tapioca starch, organic potato starch, xanthan (gum), organic high oleic safflower and/or sunflower oil, organic unsweetened cocoa powder, organic apple cider vinegar, baking soda, organic vanilla extract, sea salt.

This dessert was marketed as organic. Organic is better, but it doesn't mean healthy. If cravings for sweets are a problem for you, sometimes indulging is the key. It's about lessening the amount and consistent improvements over time that make these indulgences dissipate. Relying on fruits, honey, and maple syrup are more natural ways to handle sweetening a meal or a dessert. However, you really must understand that sugar is sugar is sugar, so they still should be used sparingly.

Allergies, Fads, and Different Diets

When I started New Life, I had to decide what kind of cuisine or food plan that I was going to provide. I considered fasting and the high-fat, protein approach, and I settled on the water-based approach to create a food cuisine that I have not changed for forty years. But in the last forty years, I have had to deal with all kinds of allergies (that have come and gone), diet plans, and food fads. For forty years the biggest expense in the New Life food plan has been produce. Our food plan gives you enough real food to do the hiking and exercises at New Life and to feel healthy in both body and mind. In our food plan, we use a very small number of products from the middle part of the grocery store.

When you fill out our New Life check-in questionnaire, we ask about any food restrictions. Some people do have very real allergies. I have learned that most others are following the latest food fad. The gluten allergy is an example of a very real allergy concern that turned into a fad. Those who truly had the allergy had to ask to not have wheat. I watched this transition occur over a three-season span. At its peak I was going through about a case of gluten-free bread a week. Within three years I was only using one a month. It was an amazing transformation to watch.

However, not one guest wrote on their questionnaires that they were allergic to enriched flour, cottonseed oil, high fructose, dextrose, yellow dye #7, and all the other words on ingredient lists that I don't understand. Please spend time looking at labels.

In effect, we are all allergic to the large volume of sugar, fat, and salt in the food products consumed. After a few days at New Life, eating tasty food transforms taste buds and creates a miracle cure for perceived allergies. That is another dimension of *authentic wellness.*

The genuine gluten allergy combined with its fad version is only one of many that have come and gone in the last forty years of food preferences at New Life. This focus on specific foods or ingredients stands in stark contrast to the central message of this book, namely that the real obstacles for almost all seeking to change food habits and become healthier are the product choices in the middle part of the grocery store, convenience stores, fast food, most restaurants, and most generally, the commercial food environments that serve unhealthy food.

There are all the different diet plans from paleo to vegetarian to vegan to whatever seems to be the diet plan that year. Some say we should eat like cavemen from prehistoric times. Others say we should be vegetarian or vegan, or they claim diet depends on blood type. However, I say that we are living in the twenty-first century with grocery stores that sell food that is not food at all and that has little or no benefit for our bodies. Learn about the foods we talk about in this book and get as much of them in your body as you can. Remember, as you make this transition, it is about the kind of food you eat, not the amount. I know that from your relationship with institutional dieting, this might not make sense to you, but from an *authentic wellness* perspective, it does. In the beginning of making a change to authentic wellness, the idea that it is not how much but what you eat can seem like a counterintuitive mind-set.

Kitchen Suggestions

One of the most common interests during my lectures involves New Life recipes. Guests are curious about recipes that are convenient enough to be done at home. In responding, I take the opportunity to go into the nuts and bolts of food-related essentials at home. First, get a nice cutting board and some decent ceramic knives. You can spend $25 on these, and you will use them for a year or two. Then if needed, buy another. You should have usable pots and pans for preparing meals. Some of these basic culinary tools have gone forgotten and unused because of the huge emphasis our culture places on convenience.

As far as recipes go, the simplest is a stir fry. It is easy to make these days with our access to the grocery store's salad bars or pre-cut vegetables. Purchase your favorite mixture of broccoli, carrots, onions, and other veggies with six to eight ounces of chicken, beef, shrimp, salmon or other sources of protein like tempeh or tofu for vegetarians. These may already be cut up and prepared by the store. If not, slice your items, place in the pan, put in a little bit of olive oil, and start sautéing. Add a tablespoon of tamari or soy sauce, a little bit of wine if you desire, and your favorite herbs. You will have yourself a healthy and beautiful stir fry. It's uncomplicated, takes very little effort, and gives you healthy water-based foods. If you are still stuck on going on a diet, have a stir fry every day for a week and call it the stir-fry diet. It will make your pond very happy.

Blenders and rice cookers are wonderful tools for our use. You can put healthy brown rice in a cooker and forget about it until mealtime. You can make shakes with bananas, frozen berries, chia seeds, kale, and other healthy ingredients. These can nourish you on the go, whether you are on the way to work or need a quick fix before you go to that cocktail party with all the unhealthy foods. Some people may worry about the additional sugars from all these fruits, but show me one person who has increased girth circumference from eating fruit. Instead the genuine concern in our culture is putting real food into our bodies. Foods that cause our problems are not going to go into a shake.

If you can, maximize the use of your time by preparing extra meals when you are cooking. Keep the food in containers for freshness. Start with seasonings and flavors that you are already familiar with and like. Then experiment and branch out. Try the seasonings used in recipes that you read and might enjoy. As your inspiration takes hold, don't forget the wine, vinegar, and basic spices that will enhance and complement your creations.

As you may have noted, this section does not provide New Life recipes as they come from our kitchen. The recipes for the meals served at New Life consist of more than 150 ingredients during a week, and they are prepared by professional chefs in a thoroughly equipped kitchen that is in constant operation from 7:00 a.m. until 8:00 p.m. Although all the New Life staff and I welcome your appreciation of the quality of our food and its service, the recipes would be of little practical use to guests at home. *Authentic wellness* means that you must find the recipes that conform to your needs and tastes and your lifestyle.

Ceramic Knife

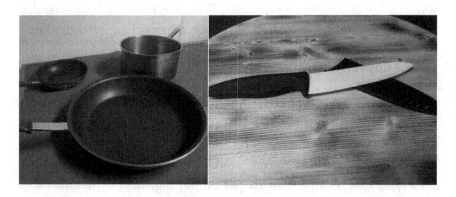

When I was a cook in the 1970s, I had the best knives money could buy. Regardless of the quality, they got dull and needed to be sharpened about once a week. It was a big hassle. Today at New Life, I have a knife company that comes once a week and brings the cooks already sharpened knives. If you do not have time to sharpen expense knives or hire someone to sharpen your knives, I have another recommendation—a ceramic knife. This is what I use at home during the off-season of New Life. They cost about $20 to $25, and if you do not drop it, they stay sharp about a year. After a year, buy another one for $25. They do come in several sizes for your cooking convenience.

Pots, Pans, and Other Kitchen Items

The three pans shown will well equip a basic kitchen for your cooking needs. The ten- to twelve-inch sauté pan is large enough for you to make a stir fry and cook other vegetables. The smaller omelet-size pan is for cooking eggs, making crepes, and putting together meals when you might be eating alone. In my opinion, you should have nonstick pans. The price for these pans should be in the middle range, not the least expensive but not the most expensive.

You will need a set of plastic utensils so that you don't damage the bottom of these pans. You can use small amounts of olive oil or butter to sauté. Another trick is to have a garden spray bottle with olive oil for sautéing. It is a healthy oil for your pond. For omelets and crepes, you can use the commercial spray cans if you wish. They are not the best, but they're okay. The pot is used for making pasta. You could also use it with a vegetable basket to steam vegetables. With a vegetable peeler, a colander, a can opener, and some small sheet pans, you have a basic kitchen setup.

Recipe Conversions

Of course, you would like to enjoy your favorite casserole or your grandmother's oatmeal cookies. Is there any way to make your favorite recipes healthy? Yes, there is. Just about any recipe that exists can be adapted to the guidelines I recommend. It's not hard to adapt a recipe, and it's a good idea because most recipes call for ingredients you now know you should avoid or limit. Even the recipes in natural foods cookbooks are not perfect. The people who wrote those cookbooks were experimenting, trying new tastes and textures.

When I (or you) adapt a recipe, our main goal is to cut down on sugar, fat, and salt. That means using 1 to 2 percent low-fat milk instead of whole milk or using plain yogurt or low-fat cottage cheese instead of mayonnaise, cream, or sour cream. You can also use half yogurt and half mayonnaise, cream, or sour cream. Take your favorite creamy salad dressing and mix half dressing and half plain yogurt for a healthy and tasty dressing, though it might take a few tries to get used to it. Sauté with small amounts of butter and olive oil. Don't use anything hydrogenated. I've never understood margarine.

Don't worry that these changes will adversely affect a recipe. They won't. What you cook will not be too dry. Nor will it fall apart. It will just be less fatty and have less sugar. Even if it doesn't seem like enough oil or fat, you can flavor the dish to taste. Over time your taste buds will change.

There are other substitutions I often make that don't have to do with fat specifically but with using healthier or less refined products.

- Use whole wheat pastry flour instead of white flour.

- Use whole grain bread. If the label says enriched flour, don't buy it.

- There is also one major rule. Don't change the proportions of baking powder and baking soda in any recipe.

The recipes listed are to teach you how to conversion recipes. They do not have enough information to be prepared and cooked. They are guides to modifying your relationship with recipes.

You can try out other ideas too. Once you get started, you'll find yourself making all sorts of creative changes. Here are a few examples. First, let's consider an oatmeal cookie recipe from a natural foods cookbook and how we modified it.

Original	New Life
½ cup butter	¼ cup butter
¾ cup brown sugar	¼ cup brown sugar
1 egg slightly beaten	1 egg slightly beaten
1 ½ tsp vanilla	1 ½ tsp vanilla
½ tsp salt	-
½ cup enriched flour	½ cup whole wheat
¾ tsp baking powder	¾ tsp baking powder
1 cup, chia seeds, ground flax seeds combo	1 cup, chia seeds, ground flax seeds combo
1 ½ cups rolled oats	1 ½ cups rolled oats
¾ cup raisins	¾ cup raisins
½ cup toasted sunflower seeds or nuts	½ cup seeds or nuts

As you see, we cut the amount of butter in half. I have experimented. It will work. We cut the amount of brown sugar by two-thirds. The cookies won't be quite as sweet, but after a few times, you won't notice. You get a good bit of natural sweeter from the raisins, or you could use chocolate chips if you're making them for your kids. A rather new product is chocolate chips with 60 percent or more cocoa. It has enough sugar flavor with less sugar. This will help your taste buds change over time. Once I tried doing 90 percent cocoa in a cookie during a play date. One kid spit out the cookie. That is why these changes are a process and very subjective. I like this kind of recipe because it has less flour and more oats. Notice this recipe can also use chia seeds, ground flax seeds, or wheat germ. This adds powerful nutritional value and doesn't really change the taste. You might also add a teaspoon of cinnamon, nutmeg, and/or clove if you wish.

Now how about trying a chicken dish? Let's consider a chicken stir fry.

Original	New Life
4 chicken breasts cut into bite size pieces	4 chicken breasts bite size pieces
2 tbsp soy sauce or tamari	2 tbsp soy sauce or tamari
½ cup olive oil	¼ cup of olive oil
2 onions chopped	2 onions chopped
2 crushed garlic cloves or	2 crushed garlic cloves
1 tsp thyme, oregano or mixed Italian herbs	1 tsp thyme, oregano or mixed Italian herbs
¼ cup dry white wine	½ cup dry white wine
Sprigs of parsley	Sprigs of parsley
1 cup chicken stock	1 cup water
2 cups Italian-style tomatoes	2 cups Italian-style tomatoes
1 lb. sliced mushrooms	1 lb. sliced mushrooms add one red diced pepper
Juice of 1 lemon	Juice of 1 lemon
1 cup pitted black olives	½ cup pitted black olives

This is very basic recipe to have stir-fried vegetable with chicken, beef, tofu, or pork. This can be served with quinoa, brown rice from the rice maker, or even the brown rice that comes in the packet from the grocery store. Instead of cooking the packet in the microwave, if you have the time, cook it in a small pan with a bit of water.

Start with olive oil in a good medium-size pan. Sauté the onions. Add the soy sauce. This will brown the onions and creates what I call a New Life roux. Like a classic French roux of butter and flour, this is the basis of any recipe that calls for a roux or sautéed onions as a start. While I was cooking at institutional kitchens, I learned that onions have so many flavors. Onions will enhance the soy sauce and give flavor. If you just added a bit of salt, you would not get the rich tamari flavor that serves as the basis for New Life soups and sautéed items. For color and nutrition, you could also add a cup of red pepper, zucchini, or summer squash. Or maybe add some leftover vegetables. With the New Life roux, you do not need salty stock. At New Life, we make a vegetable stock with all the vegetables scraps. That would be hard for you to do if time and amount were issues. You can add herbs and species, and if needed, you can also add a pinch of unprocessed sea salt.

Here's a recipe for braised fish from a low-fat, low-cholesterol cookbook.

Original	New Life
¼ cup oil	New life roux
1 ½ lbs. pan dressed fish or 1 lb. firm fish fillets such as haddock.	1 lb. firm fish fillets such as haddock
Flour	Whole wheat flour
1 tbsp. sugar	1 tbsp. orange juice
½ tsp. ginger	½ tsp. ginger
¼ tsp. garlic powder or 1 clove garlic, minced	¼ tsp. garlic powder or 1 clove garlic, minced
1 tbsp. soy sauce	1 tbsp. soy sauce
1 tbsp. sherry	1 tbsp sherry
½ tsp freshly milled black pepper	½ tsp freshly milled black pepper
Chives or green ends of spring onions	Chives or green ends of spring onions
2 medium tomatoes, chopped	2 medium tomatoes, chopped
1 tbsp. chopped parsley	1 tbsp. chopped parsley
1 tsp corn starch	1 tsp corn starch or arrowroot
½ cup water	½ cup water
Salt	-

This one for "baked potatoes stuffed with vegetables" still needs a bit of modification.

Original	New Life
4 baked potatoes	4 baked potatoes
1 cup white sauce	1 cup cottage cheese
¼ tsp salt	-
¼ cup grated hard cheese	¼ cup grated hard cheese
½ cup cooked peas	½ cup cooked peas
½ cup cooked chopped carrots	½ cup cooked chopped carrots
¼ cup diced green peppers	¼ cup diced green peppers
2 tbs diced pimientos	2 tbs diced pimientos
Au gratin	Crushed ak-mak crackers

The white sauce this recipe calls for is basically the standard roux. In this case, the white sauce is being used to bind together the vegetables and should be rather thick. Therefore, I substitute cottage cheese, which, mashed with the potato and vegetables, will achieve the desired result. Au gratin is just bread crumbs and butter, so I substitute crushed ak-mak crackers and either leave out the butter or use a very little just for flavor. Think of butter as a condiment.

Next is a recipe for a "Brussels sprout and squash casserole."

Original	New Life
1 lbs. Brussels sprouts	1 lbs. Brussels sprouts
1 ½ cups cubed winter squash	1 ½ cups cubed winter squash
1 medium onion, minced	1 medium onion, minced
1 cup chopped celery	1 cup chopped celery
¼ cup margarine	1 tbs butter
¼ cup whole wheat flour	¼ cup whole wheat flour
2 cups milk	2 cups low fat milk
½ tsp salt	-
Pepper	Pepper
Dash nutmeg	Dash nutmeg

Now let's look at a recipe for "honey cream dressing."

Original	New Life
2 eggs	2 eggs
½ cup honey	¼ cup honey
½ cup lemon juice	½ cup lemon juice
¼ cup orange juice	¼ cup orange juice
1/8 tsp sea salt	-
½ cup heavy cream	½ cup yogurt or pureed low-fat cottage cheese
2 tsp grated orange rind	2 tsp grated orange rind
Unsweetened flaked or shredded coconut	Unsweetened flaked or shredded coconut

In this case, I'd use only half the honey (taste to make sure it's okay), and instead of cream, I'd use yogurt or low-fat cottage cheese. When cottage cheese is pureed to remove the lumps, its consistency is very much like that of sour cream. The recipe is already tart. So yogurt will not be a jarring taste, but you could cut down on the lemon juice to be sure it won't be too tart.

Finally, here's a carrot cake recipe.

Original	New Life
1 ½ cup melted butter	½ cup melted butter
1 ¾ cups brown sugar or 1 ½ cups honey	¼ cup brown sugar with ½ cup honey or ¾ cup honey
4 eggs	4 eggs
3 tsp vanilla extract	3 tsp vanilla extract
Grated rind of 1 lemon	Grated rind of 1 lemon
2 cups whole wheat flour	3 ½ cups whole wheat pastry flour
2 cups white flour	½ cup of combination of chia seeds hemp seeds, sesame seeds
1 tsp salt	-
½ tsp baking soda	½ tsp baking soda
3 tsp baking powder	3 tsp baking powder
1 tsp ground allspice	1 tsp ground allspice
2 tsp ground cinnamon	2 tsp ground cinnamon

2 ½ cups packed, finely shredded carrot, soaked in juice of 1 lemon	2 ½ cups packed, finely shredded carrot, soaked in juice of 1 lemon
Optional: ¾ cup each currants or nuts	Optional: ¾ cup currants or nuts

In this recipe, I decreased the butter and sugar and specified *pastry* flour.

As you can see, converting recipes is not hard to do. It just takes a little knowledge, common sense, and a dash of creativity. Still, you've seen that you can convert any recipe with the New Life way.

I have a few more tips here.

- If you feel a recipe needs more spices or herbs to make up for omitted salt or butter, check out the internet for spice and herb options. That way, you can see what the appropriate spices are. Then add those spices to your recipe.

- Use plain yogurt as a dessert topping on fruit or dessert bread or whatever. Add a bit of orange juice or pure maple syrup to it to make it sweeter and give it extra pizzazz.

- Create a mixture of chia seeds, hemp seeds, and nibs in a container. Every day I try to have this mixture with blueberries and plain yogurt with a little maple syrup. You can add nuts or frozen fruit.

- Puree low-fat cottage cheese in a blender and substitute it for sour cream.

No doubt you'll think of more tricks as you get used to cooking this way. Maybe now you'd like to try a few conversions on your own. Here are four recipes. The way I would adapt them is shown at the end. Write your modifications in your book or on a separate piece of paper.

Stuffed Chicken Breasts	
Original	**Write Your Recipe Here.**
A boned, skinned breast of chicken.	
1 ½–2 tbs butter	

1 thin slice Virginia ham	
1 thin small piece Swiss cheese	
1 preserved kumquat or cooked apricot, sliced in half	
1 tbs finely minced shallots	
3 mushroom caps	
¼ cup dry white wine	
2 tbs freshly skinned, chopped seeded tomato	
2 tbs cream	
1 tbs parsley	

Broccoli Mushroom Noodle Casserole	
Original	**Write Your Recipe Here.**
2 stalks fresh broccoli	
1 lb fresh mushrooms	
1 large onion	
Salt and pepper	
¼ cup dry white wine	
3 eggs	
3 cups ricotta or cottage cheese	
1 cup sour cream	
3 cups wide flat egg noodles	
2 tbs wheat germ or ¼ cup bread crumbs	
1 cup grated sharp cheddar cheese	

Scalloped Potatoes	
Original	**Write Your Recipe Here.**
3 cups pared, very thinly sliced potatoes	
1 tsp salt	
2 tbs flour	
3–6 tbs butter	
¼ cup finely chopped chives or onions	

12 anchovies or 3 sliced minced crisp bacon (reduced salt)	
¼ cup finely sliced sweet peppers	
1 ¼ cups milk or cream	
1 ¼ tsp salt	
¼ tsp paprika	
¼ tsp dry mustard	

Peanut Butter Apricot Muffins	
Original	**Write Your Recipe Here.**
½ cup whole wheat flour	
¼ cup unbleached white flour	
1 tbs wheat germ	
¼ tsp sea salt	
½ tsp baking soda	
3 tbs natural peanut butter	
1 tbs butter	
½ cup dried apricots	
Boiling water	
2 tbs blackstrap molasses	
1 egg	
½ cup buttermilk	
1 tbs raw sugar	
1/8 tsp cinnamon	

Here's how I would have modified these recipes. You may not have done the same thing, but if you got rid of fat, you're doing okay.

Stuffed Chicken Breasts	
Original	**New Life**
A boned, skinned breast of chicken.	A boned, skinned breast of chicken.
1 ½–2 tbs butter	1 tbs butter or olive oil
1 thin slice Virginia ham	-
1 thin small piece Swiss cheese	1 thin small piece Swiss or mozzarella cheese
1 preserved kumquat or cooked apricot, sliced in half	1 preserved kumquat or cooked apricot, sliced in half

1 tbs finely minced shallots	1 tbs finely minced shallots
3 mushroom caps	3 mushroom caps
¼ cup dry white wine	¼ cup dry white wine
2 tbs freshly skinned, chopped seeded tomato	2 tbs freshly skinned, chopped seeded tomato
2 tbs cream	1 tbs yogurt
1 tbs parsley	1 tbs parsley

Broccoli Mushroom Noodle Casserole

Original	New Life
2 stalks fresh broccoli	2 stalks fresh broccoli
1 lb fresh mushrooms	1 lb. fresh mushrooms
1 large onion	1 large onion
Salt and pepper	Pepper
¼ cup dry white wine	¼ cup dry white wine
3 eggs	3 eggs
3 cups ricotta or cottage cheese	2 cups low-fat cottage cheese
1 cup sour cream	1 cup of ricotta
3 cups wide flat egg noodles	3 cups whole wheat, spinach or artichoke pasta
2 tbs wheat germ or ¼ cup bread crumbs	2 tbs wheat germ or crushed ak-mak crackers
1 cup grated sharp cheddar cheese	½ cup grated sharp cheddar cheese

Scalloped Potatoes	
Original	New Life
3 cups pared, very thinly sliced potatoes	3 cups pared, very thinly sliced potatoes
1 tsp salt	-
2 tbs flour	2 tbs whole wheat flour
3–6 tbs butter	2 tbs butter
¼ cup finely chopped chives or onions	¼ cup finely chopped chives or onions
12 anchovies or 3 sliced minced crisp bacon (reduced salt)	-
¼ cup finely sliced sweet peppers	¼ cup finely sliced sweet peppers

1 ¼ cups milk or cream	1 ¼ cups skim milk with ½ cup powdered milk added
1 ¼ tsp salt	-
¼ tsp paprika	¼ tsp paprika
¼ tsp dry mustard	¼ tsp dry mustard

Peanut Butter Apricot Muffins	
Original	**New Life**
½ cup whole wheat flour	¾ cup whole wheat flower
¼ cup unbleached white flour	-
1 tbs wheat germ	1 tbs wheat germ
¼ tsp sea salt	-
½ tsp baking soda	½ tsp baking soda
3 tbs natural peanut butter	3 tbs natural peanut butter
1 tbs butter	-
½ cup dried apricots	½ cup dried apricots
Boiling water	Boiling water
2 tbs blackstrap molasses	1–2 tbs blackstrap molasses
1 egg	1 egg
½ cup buttermilk	½ cup buttermilk
1 tbs raw sugar	-
1/8 tsp cinnamon	1/8 tsp cinnamon

Now from looking at the recipe exercise in the section, you have seen that the goal is to reduce fat, sugar, salt, and other unhealthy ingredients. As you change your favorite recipes to create your own healthy conversions or find new recipes, the goal is make these changes in a manner that still taste appealing while your taste buds change over time. Remember, cooking is not an exact science. For that reason, I recommend gradually weaning yourself off sugar, fat, and salt. This will be different for each of you reading this book. The finished product won't have the same consistency or taste, but with practice, you will find the right balance of taste and healthy ingredients. Your pond will thank you. Your taste buds will change. I have been working this process by developing the meal plan for New Life as well as cooking for my family.

I hope I haven't made healthy cooking sound too difficult. It's just the same as any cooking, except you begin to limit the amount of sugar, fat, and salt. Once you make a few dishes, you'll know how easy it is, even if you're a person who doesn't usually cook much. Keep in mind your motivation to cook. You can't get this food out there in the world. The only way to maintain a healthy lifestyle is to cook for yourself at least some of the time.

Recipes—Jimmy's Favorites

Although guests request New Life recipes all the time for many different reasons, I have been reluctant to share them. As you have seen, I believe that New Life recipes are less important to your lifestyle changes than for you to know how to make the healthiest food selections when ordering from a menu and how to convert recipes of your own to the healthiest versions with which you are comfortable.

I have mentioned earlier that New Life water-based recipes are skillfully prepared to assure a dining experience that pleases our guests. Over the course of a week, this requires about 150 different ingredients and professional staff working across shifts from 7:00 a.m. until 8:00 p.m. daily for twenty consecutive weeks to accomplish the ordering, receiving, storage, preparation, dining setup, meal service, and cleanup after the meals. The recipes prepared and served to guests are a product that cannot be duplicated in a home kitchen. It is unlikely, for example, that your daily dining occurs at a table for eight before, in between, or after almost constant activity. New Life's dining and activity occur in a total context that also relieves guests of a host of daily tedium that otherwise crowd life.

The total context of your ongoing existence is distinct to you alone as well. The only aspect of your ongoing daily life shared with everyone else is this very uniqueness. In this sense, the circumstances and demands of your life are subjective. They are specifically personal to you and the way you live your lifestyle. Some people work nine-to-five Monday through Friday. Others work rotating shifts or ten- to twelve-hour shifts over three or four days. Some people cook or want to learn, and some don't. Some just don't have time to cook or to learn how. Households number from a single person to any number of members. Age, gender, finances, health, physical activity, location, climate, and an endless number of other factors determine lifestyle.

For twenty consecutive weeks per year, I put my heart and soul into

New Life. Aside from an occasional family meal at home, I take frequent but brief opportunities to eat, usually standing. This grazing style is not, of course, optimal, but the food I eat is healthy. When I was a young cook, I grazed too. But forty years of grazing on the high-fat and high-sodium cuisine from institutional kitchens would create a very unhealthy pond. As of present, I am on no medications and still work ten to twelve hours most days at New Life. I attribute my well-being to my primary recommendations to you. Even though the world makes it difficult, learn to identify and consume real, water-based food.

Again, in understanding of your own lifestyle, you must determine the best route to *authentic wellness* for yourself. Every book I've ever read on some sort of diet or change in eating habits had a bunch of recipes. Recipes, like diets, are directive and prescriptive. They give the illusion of the certainty of a one-size-fits-all mentality that is impersonal, objective, and inconsistent with the reality of all our lifestyles. Accordingly, at the root of my reluctance to provide New Life recipes is, as discussed previously, the absence of the conditions necessary in your home kitchen to replicate New Life recipes and the illusion of certainty that the recipes could be mimicked in the false belief that the recipes could be your yellow brick road to *authentic wellness*.

Here are a couple of recipes I use at home. In doing so, rather than merely listing ingredients and instructions, I want to add to my presentation of the recipes an explanation about how each changed over time. I hope that this added dimension illustrates how you, too, may nurture and personalize your own favorite recipes over time so that you can improvise based on changes occurring in your lifestyle.

Here's one of my classic recipes and how it evolved. It's called Palatschinken, which is an Austrian crepe. As a cook at the hotel The Liftline Lodge, where I started New Life, the owners, Herb and Gretel Schachinger, and a Vermont chef named Charley Valentine taught me much about cooking Austrian and American cuisine.

Palatschinken was the traditional New Year's dessert. We would make more than a hundred every New Year's. This was the original recipe.

> ½ cup of enriched white flour
> ¾ cup of whole milk
> 1 egg

You put the flour in the bowl, add the milk and egg, and stir. The mixture should be a consistency of a thin milkshake.

Hint: Always pour the liquid ingredients over the dry ingredients. I made the crepes along with a dinner of beef Wellington for more than a hundred New Year's guests for four winters. My job was usually making the crepes and liver pate. (I do like liver with onions, which has both healthy and unhealthy benefits.) Use a nonstick omelet pan, and some sort of spray oil. Heat the pan up a bit. Use the spray, and then use a four-ounce ladle with the mixture. Let it cook brown on one side and flip it over.

When I started New Life, I wanted to have a Palatschinken crepe dessert, so the recipe became the following:

½ cup 100 percent whole wheat pastry flour
¾ of skim milk or 1 percent milk
2 eggs

I used 100 percent whole wheat, but whole wheat can be a bit denser than whole wheat pastry flour. However, whole wheat pastry flour is a little more difficult to find. So again, that's why there's these different trade-offs. You could use gluten-free flour as well. The mixture should have the consistency of a thin milkshake.

When I first started doing this, I would only use the egg whites, but I've came to truly believe that eggs are not an issue. They are nutritional powerhouses (for rich and poor). In my opinion, it is very rare for anyone to have health issues because they've been eating some egg yolks. It is another real food myth that takes a healthy food and trashes it without cause. Serving eggs and other hidden nutritional products is a great strategy for you and your family.

Over time I added chia seeds, hemp seeds, and even some protein powder to boost up the health benefits. When I would make Palatschinken for the family, I would four times the recipe, and one-quarter of the flour measurement would be a mixture of all these different types of seeds and powder. And I would also make enough for each family member to have two or maybe three crepes with some left over for snacks.

So now we come to the filling. In the original recipe when I started New Life, we would use a tablespoon of jam, squeeze a little lemon juice over the top, and garnish it with a bit of cinnamon.

But as it evolved, we would mix plain yogurt, no sugar cocoa powder, and maple syrup to make a thick filling and add some fresh blueberries. That is our family favorite, but the filling possibilities are endless.

You can see how a recipe evolves depending where you are in understanding your health and your cooking skills.

Oatmeal Pancakes

When I first started New Life, I would cook different breakfast option. However, I was always looking for a pancake recipe that I felt would offer the solid nutrients. I found one I liked that has flour and more oatmeal. This was the original recipe.

> ½ cup of 100 percent whole wheat flour
> 1 ½ cups of rolled oats
> 1 ½ cup of low fat or almond milk
> 2 eggs
> 2 tsp molasses, honey, or maple syrup
> 1 tbs of baking powder

This recipe makes about four to five medium pancakes. Mix flour, oats, baking powder into one bowl, and mix milk, eggs, and molasses in another. Pour the wet ingredients on the dry ones and stir until blended. You do not want the mixture to be soupy, and if you wait a few minutes, the oats will absorb the milk. You might have to add a little more milk or water because the oats will absorb the milk. This mixture should be around the consistency of a thick milkshake.

Creating food for eating in the twenty-first century is more an art than a science, and you can create options based on your time, cost, and place. In this recipe the possibilities are limitless. With the flour, for example, you can add chia seeds, cocoa nibs, and/or hemp protein. Add blueberries, strawberries, walnuts, or even chocolate chips.

Also, here's a little hint about the baking powder. You can make these pancakes four times a recipe, and I'd say for every four times, you can take off one tablespoon of the baking powder.

Make extras, refrigerate, and then put them in the toaster to make a snack.

Nuts: The Healthy Alternative to Health Bars

Although they are called health bars, almost all that are marketed are not healthy for you. While I participated at the Pritikin Institute in 2010, someone asked a very interesting question. Why was there no Pritikin bar available as a snack product? The answer was that such a product did not exist because it was not possible to create a bar with ingredient that would conform to the Pritikin food philosophy.

My own examination of many so-called health bar products on the market indicated that one of the first three labeled ingredients was always some form of sugar. The ingredient might be a harsh sugar like corn syrup, white sugar, or dextrose or one of the more exotic sugars such as honey and maple syrup.

The predominance of the sugar ingredient recalls a great quote in *Laurel's Kitchen*, a classic vegetarian cookbook by Laurel Robertson that was published in 1977, the year I went to the yoga retreat. Laurel said, "Sugar is sugar is sugar." The pertinence of that quote has become increasingly valid as additional forms of refined sugar are developed and more products with sugar as the principle ingredient become woven into what you eat. When you are reading the labels of products, be sure to note how sugar is in almost everything with a label—bacon, ketchup, beans, cereal, bread, crackers, canned fruit, vegetables, and on and on and on.

Another classic book that had a profound effect on me was *Sugar Blues* by William Duffy, which was published in 1975. It was a true eye-opener for me. Duffy presented a history of sugar to make the case that sugar consumption had become an addiction. His discussion continued and addressed the addiction. There is an accessible YouTube documentary titled *Sugar Blues* related to the book. Sugar has become so integral to our food culture that there is practically no elimination possible. However, the more you include water-based foods in your eating, the cleaner your pond becomes, which creates less desire for sugar.

When you go onto one of the many diet programs, health bars are commonly included. As mentioned earlier, you must look at the ingredients. The health bars are cheap to produce. That is why so many diet fads and diet proponents get on the so-called health bar bandwagon. There's big money to be made. Instead, let's look at a healthy alternative to the sugar-laden commercial health bars. That alternative is nuts. Nuts can be pricey, and they come with a high fat content. But nuts are a real food that will create positive results for the health of your pond.

More to the point, a healthy bag of nuts is preferable to the sugar-laced health bars. To that end, I give you my *nut bag recipe.*

As in the case of the other (more conventional) recipes offered in this book, the nut bag recipe considers factors such as taste, cost, and convenience. In creating my own recipe, I have pursued options that always include buying the more expensive nut varieties at the best available prices. If you have access to a big discount store, you can look in the nut sections to find bulk walnuts, almonds, pecans, cashews, and pistachios. These are the expensive nuts. You can also go to a Target, where they have bulk mixed nuts without added sugar and salt. A further option is the bulk section of a health food store. Even some grocery stores may have a bulk foods section. Buying in bulk will make these expensive nuts somewhat less costly. Maybe try the internet to find more ways of buying bulk nuts.

However, when you buy the nuts, as with all other foods you purchase, please do not forget to read the labels. The ingredients present in the nuts you buy must be noted and considered. The nuts you want have no added sugar, candy, salt, cottonseed oil, or ingredients you do not recognize or cannot pronounce. You want only the nut in its raw form. Your nut bag will have other real food too. There are also the cheaper nuts and seeds. These would include sunflower and pumpkin seeds as well as peanuts, which are best without salt. To add a bit of sweetness to your mix, get a box of raisins or dried apricots. You could also use prunes, figs, and dates, but they are a bit sticky. These dried fruits are very healthy and therefore better to have in your cupboards rather than in your nut mix. Eating these can help with sugar cravings and improve the purity of your pond.

You need a large glass or plastic container with a big opening on it. Any otherwise large container will do. Combine the expensive nuts with the less expensive seeds, raisins, and apricots. Try a handful. Adjust the proportion of the ingredients to your taste. Then get some plastic sandwich bags and fill them with the mixture. Put the bags in your pocket or purse and keep them with you. Bring a few bags to work. Curb your appetite with some of your mixture as a snack or use some before you go to a social setting or anywhere they may not have healthy food alternatives available. You will be getting the benefits of the healthy ingredients in so-called heathy bars without the added sugar and other unhealthy ingredients. Yes, this does take some effort. You decide if it is worth it to help purify your pond.

Studies and Claims

Studies and claims about your health are another part of understanding how to exam the vast range of information you are exposed to.

I have examined many studies that make claims and offer advice. Some find that fat, salt, and even sugar are health positive for our consumption. Unfortunately, I have found that most of such claims precipitate from the nonfood industries that produce and sell these products. Always look at the source of the study. I find these claims outlandish and amusing while recognizing the collateral damage that the confusion these claims causes. The media pick up on a study, and for that week you might have learned coffee is an antiaging agent or the endless claims like the following:

- Almonds cure cancer.

- Avocados are unhealthy.

- Wine is good for you.

- Wine is bad for you.

- An apple a day makes you lose weight.

All these claims are like the latest fads or institutional diets. The focus of what is good and bad comes and goes.

There are three studies I respect.

The *Framingham Heart Study* followed the wellness of families in Framingham, Massachusetts, beginning in 1948 and continuing to include the third generation of that Massachusetts town. I first learned about this study in 1977 when I was a cook at the Liftline Lodge. During that summer the resort was to host a group of doctors from the Boston area. (A detailed rendering of the importance of this event to my professional aspirations and the founding of New Life may be found in the biography.) The doctors' gathering was meant to design a program for the prevention of cardiac problems and other diseases associated with aging. The risk factors under examination for the detection phase of the program were derived from the *Framingham Heart Study*.

The other influential source for understanding degenerative diseases was launched by (my hero) Nathan Pritikin. Based on studies indicating that people in primitive cultures with primarily vegetarian lifestyles had little history of heart disease, he created a low-fat diet that was high in unrefined carbohydrates like vegetables, fruits, beans, and whole grains along with a regime of moderate aerobic exercise. Since Pritikin opened his institute, he has collected scientific data on his participants, creating many studies that have proven his claims of the healing benefits of a healthy lifestyle. To me, the Pritikin research is the gold standard of studies that have pointed out the value of water-based eating in our culture.

There is also an excellent book, The *China Study* by T. Colin Campbell, PhD, and Thomas M. Campbell II, MD. This book uses nutritional studies from different cultures and utilizes powerful scientific reasoning to explain why what we eat has such an effect on our health.

Let's make it simple. First, learn to take most studies and claims with less than a grain of salt. Then lean back into the principle guidelines of this book.

- If it is a water-based food, it is good for your pond.

- If it is a food that is not packaged, chances are that it is good for your pond.

- Recognize that changing eating habits is difficult because the underlying motivations are multidimensional.

- Recognize that changing eating habits is difficult because it is subjective—that is, the effective change will be very personal and individual. It will be appropriate only for you in the context of your lifestyle choices. Only you can discover and originate the change. You are the true and sole author of the change. That is why the change will be consistent with your *authentic wellness*.

Our Children

I have gone with my family to so many events that have involved food. Because of my awareness of healthy food, it can be so disheartening to go to these events and see what is served. At kids' get-togethers there usually are brownies, cookies, chips, hot dogs, and soda along with an array of nonfood. I see it at church socials, school events, family reunions, and so on. I am not saying that you should never have these foods. As I have illustrated in this book, it is the volume and abundance that is the issue. I have said throughout this book that the goal is to learn to navigate through these situations that are hard on your pond.

I have been fighting against unhealthy food relationships for most of my life. It has been a long battle with many small victories, and I've helped many people along the way; however, it's a battle that we're losing, and it's a battle that we just can't afford to lose. I hope that this book has helped you see that we are water-based creatures with certain food needs. I hope that it has also helped you find small incremental changes that over time can lead to improving your lifestyle. I hope that it has opened your eyes to some of the shifts that our society needs to make. That change starts with a process of personal transformation.

Takeaways

Although you are reaching the end of the book, you are at the beginning of the lifestyle changes that place you on the path to *authentic wellness*. You now have a framework in which to consider how to travel on that path. Hopefully, our discussion of the education, psychology, and sociology of eating will serve you well in perceiving the many dimensions that affect your relationship with food and your food behaviors. I hope that you understand what I have referred to interchangeably as healthy and real food and that you now have learned that personal habits and the world around you don't make it easy to navigate toward a water based being. The goal is that *authentic wellness* will help you let go of much of what you are familiar with like counting calories, weight, and dieting. This then will help you create a new perspective that will benefit you in fashioning a personalize wellness strategy that will lead you toward a successful path of quality life and longevity.

Once you have taken the first steps on your journey, your momentum forward will make you increasingly conscious of the well-being that you are experiencing. The healthy food that you eat creates a well-being that will motivate you to seek and to discover foods and forms of fitness that are compatible with your evolving lifestyle. These changes will be incremental and subjective. In short, they will be very personal. You will shed behaviors that have corralled you into food choices and actions that you now realize cannot help you attain the well-being you seek.

The mind-body connection of which we have spoken will become steadily apparent and a supporting resource to you as you progress on your own journey. As your awareness changes, so will your body and its well-being. You will deservingly derive personal satisfaction from the well-being experienced from your progress. Your path forward will not be easy because of the institutionalized roadblocks and hazards, both great and small. However, your own efforts are a contribution to an emerging societal recognition of the many health and cost issues that have arisen from the distortion of our food supply. The urgency attached to the restoration of the food supply to its water basis is clear.

Furthermore, while this book is for you, it has, of course, been a labor of love I have wanted to complete for a considerable time. For four decades New Life has given me a platform on which to share my views with our guests. This book enables me to maintain and deepen my relationships with those who have participated at New Life and to reach out to others. The book also enables me to resolve my own frustration about the impossibility—as much as I would have had it otherwise—of delivering a lecture that contained all I wanted to convey. Nonetheless, during those lectures, there were themes and concerns that arose repeatedly. Before concluding, I want to leave you with the bottom line on these topics to consider on your journey.

At the end of a lecture, I would be astonished to receive questions about the number of calories in the lentil soup or about an internet statement that suggested it was not good to mix yogurt with blueberries or about whether raw almonds and avocados were not good to eat because of too much fat. In the broadest perspective, fat from foods in their natural forms will not be harmful and are not the issue in the food supply we now have. Eat them as you wish. Eat whatever amount you wish of any water-based food from nuts, avocados, beets, real whole grains, fruit, or vegetables. Over time this will change your relationship with food and allow you to become more aware of what true hungry is. You will have a water-based body that creates health and vitality regardless of your age.

Allergies are, of course, a genuine concern and not to be treated lightly. A great variety of these have ebbed and flowed in emphasis over time. But no one—not a single person—has ever told me about an allergy to cottonseed oil, palm oil, hydrogenated oil, yellow dye #10, dextrose, and the array of unrecognizable and unpronounceable chemicals that are processed into our food. Our health would be better served by avoiding the preponderance of foods with harmful substances to which little attention is paid. To quote my own depiction of this misplaced obsession, "No one ever told me that they were allergic to a Big Mac." True allergies cannot be ignored, but our efforts at well-being would improve considerably by recognizing and not consuming the very harmful ingredients that are present in our food.

Internet blogs and magazines are not a substitute for reading the labels on food packages at the grocery store. The media, especially the institutional dieting proponents, may give direction on foods to eat or to avoid. Because fats in food are particularly prone to misunderstanding, the media may, for example, caution you not to consume avocados, walnuts, almonds, cashews, sunflower seeds, or butter. Indeed, if you are buying any of those foods in packaged form, examine the labeling carefully to avoid the negative effects on your health that cottonseed oil, palm oil, or hydrogenated oil would cause. On the other hand, even if you must spend a bit more to buy these foods without these unhealthy additives, any fats you take in as you are consuming these real foods will be less harmful to you. Again, in the broadest perspective, clogged arteries and high blood pressure have never been attributed to overeating avocados and nuts. The more you understand about your relationship with water-based food, the better you can understand information from the media as a source for nutrition education.

As we have mentioned, eggs can be a source of considerable confusion. Or more precisely, the yoke has received bad press over the years for the cholesterol concerns it raises. My veggie omelet caused me to throw away many yolks. After a while my thought about the yolk began to change. I never liked throwing out all those yokes, and as I learned about the excellent sources of protein and nutrients eggs were, I began to feel silly about it. Now I focus less on the cholesterol than on the egg as a nutrient-packed, real food that I can recommend as affordable and perhaps of special value to vegetarians.

Please understand that I am not recommending the egg if that is contrary to your doctor's advice. In relation to the egg, however, instead of fixating on it as a culprit, I am once more urging that you assess your eating habits broadly to see whether you are consuming ingredients that would be far more harmful to you than the egg. On the higher plane from which to understand how healthy you are living, try to pay heed, for example, to how much sugar you are consuming. Try to determine whether there is cottonseed oil, palm oil, or hydrogenated oil present on its own or among the other natural oils in foods you are consuming.

In this respect, I hope you see that regardless of the headlines or the blame attributed to the nutritional evils of the egg, the egg itself or any other real food could not be a health problem for you. There are, however, ingredients in food to which you may be paying no attention at all that pose real dangers to your health and well-being. Recognize that your health depends substantially on understanding the difference between real food and the other possibly very harmful substances that are incorporated into the food you eat.

A great source of authentic nutritional education can be found by subscribing to the *Nutrition Action Health letter*, the flagship publication of the Center for Science in the Public Interest (CSPI). This publication originated at about the same time as New Life began and is based in Washington, DC. I very much admire Michael F. Jacobson, PhD, cofounder and president of the CSPI. The CSPI lobbies Congress to help shape national policies on food, nutrition, wellness, and healthy eating. I have subscribed to this monthly newsletter for thirty years. I recommend it to you for its excellent coverage of food and nutrition issues and because your subscription will contribute to the CSPI's mission.

A Recipe to Implement Authentic Wellness

First ingredient: *Realize* we cannot continue as individuals and as a society to consume high volumes of nonfood. There is plenty of evidence to argue that the increase to girth circumference, the development of obesity, and the progression of degenerative diseases have reached epidemic proportions.

Second ingredients: *Convert* your knowledge of dieting, weight loss, and calories, into forming the authentic wellness mind-set that you have learned, which will contribute toward the health of your pond.

I realize there is a lot of information out there, some of which is contradictory about how to take care of your pond. There are perilous mind-sets about dieting, weight loss, and how you should look. We are oversaturated with celebrities and photo editing, which creates lofty and impossible standards of beauty. If you hold onto the old beliefs, attaching to media-driven standards about who you should be, and measure results in a linear way of immediate short-term improvements, you will stay in the mind-set of institutional dieting. Here are some of the most common things I have heard: "I want to look like I did when I was younger." "People around me want me to look a certain way." "I want to look like the media says I should." "I want to weigh a certain amount." "I have to go on a diet." You should focus on your body as a water-based being and think about how to keep your pond from the polluting food that is all around you.

Third ingredients: *Strive* toward a healthy lifestyle.

Here are a few ideas. How about striving for a healthy lifestyle so that you are not on any medications like antacids, which take the acid out of your stomach, laxatives, which are usually needed because of the lack of fiber in the nonfood you are eating, or medications taken for high blood pressure, diabetes, and other degenerative diseases. It truly is frightening the disclaimers about the dramatic side effects of these "medicines." Strive to lead a life that requires as little medication, both prescription and over-the-counter drugs, as possible. Pritikin has proven scientifically it can be done with a healthy lifestyle. This book gives you the tools to begin this journey toward a quality of life without the drug-infested solutions that are already so much a part of your lifestyle. Ask yourself how you are doing and how you can strive for a quality of life that will increase longevity, energy, and activity. Regardless of what age you are, strive toward eating water-based foods at a pace that works for you.

Enjoy the journey. Let's take care of our ponds. As we do, the pace at which we succumb to degenerative diseases will slow down, and our girth circumference will become less. Take the information from the book, and at your own pace, create new ways to change your relationship with food and your well-being. This will truly create a path to *authentic wellness*.

BIOGRAPHY

The goal of this biography is to express to you my personal journey as it relates to the people, places, ideas, influences, trends, and times I came upon over my life, including the four-decade transformation of New Life, that have helped to create what has become *authentic wellness*.

Childhood

I was born in 1950 at the cusp of the second half of the twentieth century in Stoneham, Massachusetts. The baby boom generation was in full swing, and Americans were shopping in big grocery stores. TV dinners, television, and fast food were just beginning to become a part of our culture. Nonfood, which is food that has no or little nutritional value, began to become an ever-increasing portion of our food supply.

When I was five years old, for a variety of reasons, my family first moved to Gainesville, Florida, and then over to Panama City, Florida. My father, a World War II veteran, was a carpenter, and my mother was a homemaker. I recall taking family drives back and forth between Panama City and Gainesville. Our routine provided for stopping on the route's only eating opportunity at one of the newly opened McDonald's. In the earliest McDonald's, fresh potatoes were peeled and cooked into the fries they served. The milkshakes had real milk.

At that time, even McDonald's had not fully crossed the threshold into the food-industrial complex. Over time this complex has dominated our food landscape to create an environment of unhealthy food. You may wish to view *The Founder*, a film that dramatizes the part of Ray Kroc's life related to the creation of fast food and its permeation of American cuisine and culture.

My father died when I was ten. Our family lived on social security. Without social security and my mother working a bit, I am not sure what would have happened. I got a paper route when I was thirteen. Food was a big issue. For part of the month, we had some, and during other parts we had less. This was the beginning of me learning to create food that was convenient and inexpensive but also tasted good.

Growing up in Florida to Working in Vermont Kitchens

After high school I attended a local junior college for a year and a half. My grades were good enough to earn a winter semester transfer to Florida State University in Tallahassee. When I got to Florida State, I felt that I had reached a point from which I could explore, learn, and grow in a completely different environment. I received subsidized housing from the Southern Scholarship Research Foundation. The foundation continues to grant low-cost housing and food to qualified students. We had an allotment of food for breakfast, lunch, and dinner. We took turns cooking and doing other household chores. The food was cheap, but it did get us by.

The head of the scholarship house was John Haynes, a counseling major. He introduced me to the world of therapy. I remember seeing films of a renowned Gestalt therapist of the time named Fritz Pearls. I attended therapy workshops, and from this expanded perspective, I began changing my outlook.

This was the tumultuous 1960s, which was radical in so many well-known ways. My focus will be the deep-seated transformation that I experienced and participated in related to food, fitness, and overall wellness. My earliest exposure to this phenomenon was a food co-op in the basement of a Seventh-day Adventist Church. There, I learned about eating peanut butter without sugar, 100 percent whole wheat flour, brown rice and granola. There, people bought healthy food in bulk. Although I could not know then, this was the infancy of the health food stores that would sprout up all over the country.

Vegetarian cuisine gained popularity. *Diet for a Small Planet* (1971) by Frances Moore Lappé became a best seller. It was the first major book to cite the environmental impact of meat production as wasteful and a contributor to global food scarcity. She argued for environmental vegetarianism, which meant choosing what was best for the earth and our bodies—a daily action that reminds us of our power to create a saner world. More generally, the book represented one element of the countercultural transformation during that period.

Another characteristic of the food, fitness, and overall wellness transformation of the time was dieting. The Scarsdale diet may have been the most prevalently publicized of the period. Of course, there were many others then, with many more to come. I can tell you that dieting never made sense to me despite my motivation to live a healthy lifestyle. My preference was to eat good food and stay active. However, because the concept of dieting became so pervasive in American life, my professional dedication to *authentic wellness* compelled me to remain in constant disagreement with the idea and practice of dieting.

At Florida State, I majored in social studies education. The coursework introduced me to geography, sociology, anthropology, political science, history, and education. The undergraduate portion of my formal education occurred during a time when the education process was itself experiencing a radical transformation. During this time, educator John C. Holt wrote the first of his many books, *How Children Fail* (1964), to decry schools designed for the industrial revolution and to call for a classroom environment in which students would feel more comfortable and confident. *Summerhill: A Radical Approach to Child Rearing* (1960) is a book about Summerhill's School, an educational environment that called for a "free school" with no classroom or curriculum.

This type of thinking prepared me to look beyond the boundaries of the strictly academic edges of these subject areas. My generalist education was instrumental in finding knowledge and information that formed the underlying patterns, trends, and connections among these disciplines. Over time I began to see the world in dimensions not governed by categories and divisions. We will understand later how my generalist mode of thought pertains to nutrition and fitness. For the moment, I recall a realization of this transformation that struck me while I was still an undergraduate.

My student loans required that I work as much as I could. The campus computer building's very large room housed the mammoth machines of that time. I worked an overnight shift. I fed the IBM punch cards into the machines that devoured them to keep operating. Even at that early point in data processing, I was struck by the advancements in technological expertise required for these computers to function. I was amazed by how far technology had come, but at the same time, our ability to feed ourselves wisely enough to maintain our health didn't seem to give people a workable strategy to create a healthy lifestyle in a dramatically changing culture.

After graduation from Florida State, my burning desire was to head north. In Schenectady, New York, I visited with my sister, Patty, and her husband, Fred, as I hunted for a teaching position. I knew that teaching jobs at that time were very scarce, and I took an interview in Wilmington, Vermont. During the interview I noticed a very discouraging stack of resumes on the interviewer's desk. This made me open to suggestions about jobs at Vermont ski resorts. I went to the Snow Lake Lodge at Mount Snow, Vermont, and they offered me a job washing dishes or making salads and desserts. As a college graduate, I decided on making salads and desserts.

As it happened, this job was just right for me. I worked with a very accomplished executive chef named Tommy Mencheck, who was a graduate of the Culinary Institute, a French chef named Jackie, and a local Vermonter named Chuck.

I made $50 per week with room and board, and I also received a ski pass. Skiing was the highlight of my day. I was a cooking ski bum. I worked and skied hard. It was a very comfortable and earnest working environment. And for better or worse, I had enough to eat. I was always picking on desserts, prime rib, and the rest of the staples and delicacies in the hotel's food panorama, complete with all the unavoidable sugar, fat, and salt. This was the beginning of my life in Vermont. I have spent every summer ever since involved in the operation of a hundred-room hotel in the Green Mountains.

After a year I moved to Stratton, Vermont, where I worked at the Stratton Mountain Inn. There, I took lessons from Austrian ski instructors, and in the summer I played tennis. In the year I was there, I worked behind the range, where I enhanced my cooking skills by learning to make prime rib, beef wellington, hollandaise sauce, and other sophisticated dining fares. These formative experiences were the foundation of a life in the realms of food (if not yet nutrition), exercise (if only for myself), and hard work. The seasonal nature of the work also gave me an off-season opportunity to explore other places.

In my second year at Stratton, I moved next door to the Lifeline Lodge. It was owned by an Austrian couple, Herbie and Gretel Schachinger. Their families had run resorts for generations in Austria. From the Schachingers, especially Herbie, I learned a lot about entrepreneurship. In the kitchen Charlie Ballentine, a local Vermont chef, helped me with my culinary proficiencies in both American and Austrian cuisines. We worked together preparing a wide range of dishes from frog legs to wiener schnitzel and dumplings. But the intensity of cooking into the evening left only the evening hours for me to relax. Occasionally, I would socialize at the hotel bar. The bar was not a real lure for me because I was never a drinker despite my exposure to alcohol. As in childhood, my ten-o'clock retreat to the comfort of television and my habit of eating unhealthy food late at night was more my preference.

It was not that I did not know that the unhealthy late-night eating was a problem, but I did become more thoughtfully focused on it than ever before. But the dilemma before me was the difficulty of somehow eating earlier when confronted with the stress of cranking out a hundred dinners. I coped with but did not satisfy my hunger during the cooking. I would graze in the kitchen. To cope with my hunger and to enjoy my food with a degree of relaxation, I continued reluctantly to succumb to unhealthy late-night eating. Still, I could not overcome the sense that there must be some way to change my unhealthy eating behavior.

Consequently, along with the other changes presented by my Vermont life, there was an emerging recognition of the complexities of my own relationship to food and eating behavior. This insight caused me to realize that eating behavior had dimensions of which we could be aware and at least some of which we were apparently unaware. Until I became aware of those dimensions of my eating habits that were not evident to me, it would be difficult to make choices about alternatives that might liberate me so that I might act in a healthier manner.

Let the Off-Season Traveling Begin

In 1975, during a fall break from cooking, I embarked on a six-week trip to Europe. My itinerary started in Amsterdam and took me to the Mona Lisa in Paris, Goya in Spain, a mutual friend in Morocco, Rome, Innsbruck (to experience Herbie and Gretel's hometown), skiing in Switzerland, and back to Amsterdam. Europe did not have the packaged food that was typical of the middle aisles in the American grocery store.

Europeans appeared to eat primarily when hungry and did so together in a relaxed manner.

Back from Europe with a new perspective, I realized my relationship with food was changing. The tension between who I was as a cook in Herbie's kitchen and who I might become heightened further as I traveled to Montreal, Nova Scotia, Boston, and the New England area. I began to feel that I had learned as much as I could from Herbie, Gretel, and Charlie. I came to realize that my life required a change.

At that time, to channel my need for change, I attended a local yoga class. My need to do this was, in part, prompted by my concern that my health was impacted in a negative way. In fact, I was close to being addicted to cigarettes. A cook in need of a break who appears to be standing around is "lazy." But a cook smoking a cigarette is on a genuine break. The more I stayed around prime rib, schnitzel, and dumplings, the more I began to feel that I was stuck in a life that was unhealthy.

As I continued yoga, I was beginning to cook brown rice for myself and to explore health food stores for healthier eating alternatives. I found out about a yoga retreat in the Laurentian Mountains, north of Montréal. Since summer business at the Liftline Lodge was in the off-season, Herbie agreed I could leave for six weeks to attend the yoga retreat.

At this retreat I ate healthy food, did lots of yoga, and became a certified yoga instructor. I truly believe that if I had not done the retreat, I would have become addicted to cigarettes. On my very first day back at work after my six-week experience, I was cooking institutional food in the Liftline Lodge kitchen. My mind could not help but think that my life was about to take a new direction. It did.

After I got back from my yoga experience, a surprising event transpired. A group of Boston dentists owned the Liftline Lodge. Bernie Howes, one of the owners, had experienced cardiac complications. Bernie's interest in cardiac issues motivated him to develop a risk factor assessment that included a cardiac stress test and analysis of everything from exercise and eating habits to whether you wore a seatbelt. Bernie wanted to hold several summer workshops on his evaluation process at the Liftline Lodge for doctors. He wanted Herbie to provide the food.

Bernie asked Herbie to make sure that the food would be consistent with the health theme of the doctors' gathering. Herbie understood the purpose of the gathering, but he had no clue what Bernie meant by healthy food. Herbie did indicate to Bernie that he had a second chef named Jimmy who fed the staff brown rice, went to a yoga retreat, and was familiar with these kinds of things. Bernie and Herbie asked me if I could prepare an appropriate menu. I jumped at the chance and began to examine cookbooks for this project.

The challenge of healthy recipes was tough back then because very few recipes were designed to reduce sugar, salt, and fat, still taste good, and be convenient to prepare. I considered these parts of the challenge and became creative at converting recipes to make them healthier by substituting ingredients that still tasted good.

I did cooking demonstrations for Bernie's workshops. One of my best presentations gave rise to the now classic egg white omelet. Because the egg whites alone were somewhat bland, I figured we could use a single yoke with the three egg whites. I demonstrated that the addition of spinach, mushrooms, and all variety of veggies along with a bit of cheese made for a convenient and delicious entrée. I also began to include in my talks at Bernie's workshops the importance of produce and the sections of the grocery to frequent and those to avoid.

There was practically no one with whom I could share my yoga experiences. Joan Cullins, a California psychologist, found out that I had taken this yoga retreat and was curious about my experience. Joan stayed every summer at the resort with her husband, who had run the golf program. Joan and I met and discussed my yoga experience. She showed me an article in *Vogue* magazine about a wellness retreat in California called the Ashram. The article's key points were about the need to drink more water and the body-mind connection that was very much in line with what I learned from the yoga experience.

At that time, the Arnold Palmer golf program for teenagers was housed at part of the Liftline Lodge called the Glockenhoff. At the end of that summer, they were going to move the operation to another location. At the same time, Joan and I began to formulate the idea of starting a health spa. I could teach yoga while serving healthy food. Joan could do guided walks and talk about changing eating habits. In the basement of the Glockenhoff, there was a mother-daughter team, Nina and Garrett, that taught calisthenics for adult gymnastics. They, too, were interested in our plan. Quite amazingly, a health spa enterprise was coming together.

We met with Herbie, and he allowed us to use the Glockenhoff. Joan and I discussed the enterprise's mission statement and philosophy. We had to articulate these so that we could communicate clearly about our marketing strategy. My own sense of our philosophy came from how I felt when I placed *Vogue, Self,* and *GQ* on one side of the table and the *Yoga Journal* and *East/West Journal* on the other side. I remember saying that I wanted to create something in the middle. We agreed that it was going to be about creating a "new life" for people, and so we decided to name it "The New Life Health Spa." At the end of that summer, we pooled a thousand dollars each to open New Life Health Spa in the summer of 1978. A few years later it was renamed New Life Hiking Spa®.

During the winter before New Life's first season, I talked with Joan back in California after 11:00 p.m. when the phone rates were less. To promote New Life, we created a brochure. I took a bus to Manhattan to leave the brochures among the women's magazines at the reception areas at the Conde Nast Building at 350 Madison Avenue.

But most importantly, what was I going to feed people? I knew it wasn't going to be industrial kitchen food I have been trained to prepare. To answer this, I spent a lot of time reading to come up with healthy recipes. I read Pritikin's book and his ideas helped me to create an overall food philosophy. The menu would include lots of vegetables and fruits with some veal, fish, chicken, and some whole grains. I got many of my recipe ideas from the classic cookbook *The Joy of Cooking.* I used these recipes for their unique ingredients. I then made conversions to reduce or eliminate sugar, fat, and salt, which the Pritikin approach had taught me.

Early New Life

New Life was to be housed in the Glockenhoff, the thirty-room building that was one of three buildings of the hundred-room Liftline Lodge. Herbie let me use the apartment suite to operate New Life. I used the apartment kitchen to prepare the food. The living room became the dining room, and my office was the suite bedroom. The first summer of New Life, I had twelve guests. At times there was only a single guest to benefit from my yoga class and healthy meals. We had very little fitness and no hiking. Nina and Garret has calisthenics classes. My yoga class was at four o'clock, so I started cooking dinner at five o'clock. Joan would take everybody on a walk. What really mattered to guests was that they lost weight. They did.

After that first season, Joan told me that she had to leave the partnership because she and her husband would not be returning to Stratton. I went back to work for Herbie in the kitchen, but I remember that I always did something for New Life every day and began to feel the transition from the cooking to becoming an entrepreneur. I knew now that I could be healthy in the summer. Even if I went back to some of my old habits in the winter, I tried to be active and look ahead.

New Life continued in its second summer with basically the same format as the first season. I had twenty-five guests. We served very small portions. When asked, I would say that the meals were eight hundred calories, which from the guests' perspectives was fine because their main objective was weight loss. Stress reduction, wellness, and lifestyle change were not on their radar.

In society at large, there emerged an increasing focus on personal well-being that was reflected in health and fitness trends. The effects of the women's movement of the 1960s were evident as well. By the late 1970s and early 1980s, women were making deserved inroads into the workforce. This led to lifestyle stresses that a healthy getaway could accommodate.

After the second summer at New Life, many aspects of my life started to transform completely. I was an entrepreneur and sole owner of a business. I was a person beginning a dedicated exploration of an emerging revolution in fitness, nutrition, and wellness. I felt determined to absorb, participate in, and put into my own new life and New Life the most contemporary thoughts and changes in wellness. With focus and hard work, I began to see that New Life was becoming a healthy environment for my personal growth and the wellness of all involved.

During the second summer, I began to see a pattern among guests in the six-day program. I wanted to understand how the guests were experiencing New Life, while at the same time there were so many other decisions about the New Life program that I had to make. In the beginning I used exercise mats, but as low- and high-impact aerobics were getting popular, I had to make a major decision to buy a spring floor to be customized for the fitness area. I invested in copper pots and fine kitchen cutlery to maximize New Life's ability to create its healthy and tasty recipes.

After the second summer, I participated in a trade show in New York City. I came across a small marketing company called E & M Associates. It was a mother-and-daughter team, Elizabeth and Martha. Elizabeth was a retired travel editor from *Town & Country Magazine*. I paid them $150 to write me a press release to their contacts. This relationship grew to the point that when I was in New York, I could use their office. This allowed me to diversify my marketing and promotional efforts. This was before the internet.

Through the 1980s, I learned to market New Life across many venues. I appeared on Regis Philbin's local television show. There I demonstrated my signature three egg white one yoke veggie omelet. I took radio interviews in the city and the New England area. I attended regional trade shows, and lunched with newspaper and magazine health editors and reporters.

After the third season, I started to get serious press. The big break came when Diane Whitehead, the travel editor of the *Boston Globe*, came to New Life for a week. This became a two-page spread in the Sunday travel section of the *Globe*. That year New Life was listed by *Money Magazine* as one of the top ten spas in the country. It was clear that New Life was taking off.

Through all of this, guests came on Sunday and left on Saturday. Their total focus was about losing weight. Although weight loss was of little interest to me, I could see people changing in the six nights at New Life. I observed their bodies at their first yoga session, which I taught on Sunday afternoon. I was always taken by the differences that had transpired by the Friday afternoon session. At Friday night's lecture, which was titled "Life after New Life," we talked about how to realistically integrate the ideas they'd learned as New Life guests into their home lives.

I spoke about the healing effects of good food and how they might look at their home food environments and behaviors to find healthful adaptations. When I mentioned Pritikin and the idea that good food healed, there was occasionally a physician or other medical person who stated that Pritikin's claims had not been proven. Then I simply continued diplomatically rather than argue or concede. Pritikin's ideas had not been proven at that time, but they have been since. Pritikin was, indeed, a scientific pioneer whose work demonstrated that food could heal the body.

Leaving Herbie's Kitchen

After the third summer, I realized it was time to create a cycle of New Life operating in the summer and focusing on marketing in the off-season. It was time for me to leave Herbie's kitchen. I sensed this life would be healthier in mind and body and that it would allow me to explore many facets of wellness. It was always my hope that guests at New Life would figuratively be able to leave Herbie's kitchen too. I wanted guests to understand how the healthy environment I had created at New Life can go home with them.

I realized also that New Life was created for me to be in a healthy environment. It was a place for me to express how I felt about what I thought was one of the biggest problems in our country—what we eat and the effect it has on our health. At New Life, I have reached a significant amount of people to help in their pursuit toward a healthy lifestyle. For this I am very proud.

I also have felt frustrated because there was a limit to how many people I could reach. I felt that to fully understand the many aspect of changing eating habits, I needed a greater platform to help people beyond a visit to New Life. With the epidemic of degenerative disease and upsurge in girth circumference, the increased acceptance that institutional dieting is not working, and the trend toward wellness, I felt only recently it was time for me to write a book. The goal being to help even more people leave Herbie's kitchen.

If I Can Make It There

After the third season of running New Life, I left Herbie's kitchen and my career in institutional kitchens. Most winters during the 1980s, I lived in New York City, while in the spring, summer, and fall, I ran New Life. I had the added bonus that many of the guests who came to New Life were from New York City. I began to accept invitations that brought me to their offices and places of business. I was present in the city for the wellness explosion of the 1980s. I was there to witness, understand, participate in, and perhaps in a very modest way, impact the wellness revolution that took place.

The high interest rates and the endless gas station lines of the late 1970s transformed into the economic recovery of the 1980s. As women gained disposable income from their progressive integration into the workplace, men and families had to adjust to the impact of this changing lifestyle. These adjustments were complicated by the unhealthy food production and consumption that, along with sedentary lifestyles, were rooted in the 1950s.

The American marketplace responded vigorously to the health and fitness concerns that arose. A fitness industry burst upon the scene. Jane Fonda, the period's "queen of fitness," released her first VHS cassettes. There came step classes, high- and low-impact aerobics, power yoga, and genres of dance classes. Our basements and spare rooms became places filled with exercise routines and formidable fitness hardware.

As I began my marketing efforts in the city, I saw the first signs advertising the soon-to-be-opened New York Health and Racquet Club. I stopped into many Manhattan health clubs where cardiovascular and weight devices had replaced the rows of belt-driven machines that sought to wiggle the fat away. Big companies were putting fitness devices in their offices. Hotels were making the devices available to travelers. The jargon that accompanied the new devices consisted of terms like "aerobic" and "target heart rate." The overall balance of activity for fitness was becoming understood as cardiovascular, stretching, and strengthening. Massage and other forms of bodywork were acknowledged for their revitalization and healing benefits.

I updated my understanding of aerobics through the book *Fit or Fat* by Covert Bailey and a trip to the Kenneth Cooper Institute in Dallas, Texas. I had to adapt from high- to low-impact aerobics. When I started, the word aerobics was not in the general vocabulary. The classic yoga I had learned turned into what I called Western yoga. Classes like power yoga did kind of confuse me.

I had witnessed the health club boom and then joined a health club association beginning in the early 1980s. I participated in a couple of their conventions. This allowed me to observe the continuing transformation of wellness. As New Life developed in the 1980s, traditional wellness practice obligated me to weigh, measure, and take a body mass index measurement. I always felt that the fit of your clothes was a less technical assessment that made sense to me.

One indication that the overwhelming change was not all good came when I visited a show in Chicago. I came across an attendee who told me he had tested a variety of instruments that measured body mass index. His calibration results indicated that almost none of the instrument's measurements were correct. Almost every instrument yielded a significantly different measurement. By the mid-1990s, we didn't do anything but weigh guests because the wellness industry and the public remained fixated on weight loss. I needed to stay in business, so I kept my scale and weighed New Life guests. Today I have the same scale I bought in 1985. Some guests find it and weigh themselves. Guest now come for the wellness experience of New Life, and although weight loss does occur, that is not necessarily their goal or fixation.

The 1980's health explosion was the perfect storm for me and for New Life. I had the good fortune to be right there as all this reverberated and sorted itself into its various levels of true worth. Doing New Life in the summer and creating a wide range off season wellness experiences enabled me to refine and propel my personal and business aspirations toward fitness and the more encompassing realm of wellness. In the city I learned about the most effective options for fitness and wellness.

My eclectic, nonlinear approach to wellness and my opportunity to experience this wellness transformation from so many perspectives taught me to make selective distinctions from among often confusing and contradictory claims. Instead, to form a basis for *authentic wellness*, I could identify the significant interplay points among these many fitness and nutritional alternatives.

I Can Make It Anywhere

My first apartment in Manhattan was a sublet on Fourth Street and Sixth Avenue near Washington Square Park. One day I received a letter from someone named Mel Zuckerman from Tucson, Arizona.

This is how it happened. Dorothy and Carl Bennett, the original owners of the retail department store chain Caldor's, which owned over 50 retail stores at the time, had been one of the first New Life guests. Although New Life did not meet their upscale expectations, they understood and valued what I was doing at New Life. After their visit they sent me a thank-you letter saying, "To Jimmy, who is doing so much with so little."

The letter I had received in my New York apartment was from Mel Zuckerman, who with his family had recently started the Canyon Ranch Spa. Mel was a land developer who had visited the Oaks Spa in Ojai, California, because of health reasons. It was founded and run by Sheila Cluff, who is a true pioneer in the destination spa industry. Mel's incredibly positive health experience at the Oaks convinced him and his wife, Enid, to buy a rundown Tucson dude ranch. In 1978, with a large investment, the Zuckerman family established and operated a truly premier destination spa.

After leaving New Life, the Bennett's later visited the Canyon Ranch Spa. They talked with Mel, who mentioned how frustrating it was to find people who truly understood his vision of a destination wellness environment for a healthy lifestyle. They told him about me, and he tracked me down. When Mel and I got to speak by telephone, he indicated that he was working toward an association of destination spas that focused on providing life-changing health experiences. Mel invited me to come out to Tucson. I flew out for a visit.

The Canyon Ranch Spa was an extremely larger and more upscale version of what I was doing and hoped to do at New Life. Mel and I hit it off instantly. We chatted extensively about wellness philosophy and how a destination spa could help people focus on a healthy lifestyle to then continue in their lifestyle back home. Our discussion seeded an association that became the Destination Spa Group, an organization that from the late 1980s through the 1990s, served to educate consumers about the destination spa industry and the standards that a genuine spa experience should meet. This was also the beginning of a lifelong friendship with Mel and his family. This included Mel's string of twelve summer visits to New Life.

I was the Zuckerman's guest at the ranch for the winter of 1982. The ranch became a base for me to practice my own wellness, to acquire a series of experiences and perspectives on the spa industry, and to shape my own sense of the directions my life could continue to take.

From a personal and practical standpoint, my winter opportunities at the Canyon Ranch constituted the best education for understanding a destination spa operation. I soon began to realize the complexities that differentiated a business operation on the scale of Canyon Ranch from a small organization like New Life.

Still, it was clear that the personal dedication of Mel, Enid, and their family reduced the highly structured Canyon Ranch operation to a family business by their hands-on grace and presence. Mel taught me that wellness was the product of a destination spa that had "an energy source." Mel and family were that source for the ranch. He also pointed out that the entire enterprise was the success and interaction of its four essential parts—the health club, hotel, restaurant, and educational institute. Mel's perspective certainly seems borne out by the success that I saw the ranch experiencing while I was there. It was evolving into one of the most prestigious destination spas in the country. Its guests were from the top tier in wealth, exclusivity, and even celebrity. In addition to CEOs and other elites, I met James Taylor and Yoko Ono.

Mel and his family put me in touch with more profound realizations than the operation of the business. Mel's view was that a destination spa had to have an energy source, a person at its core to guide the many facets of this type of business operation. That is what you want to look for when you chose a destination spa experience to enhance your personal wellness.

During the 1980s, California was a true mecca for spa destinations. I had an opportunity to visit many of these facilities. My visits included The Oaks (previously mentioned), The Ashram in Calabasas ("boot camp of the stars"), LaCosta (resort spa) in Carlsbad, and Rancho LaPuerta (established in the mid-1940s) in Tecate, Mexico, south of San Diego. In California, there was also my favorite wellness retreat, Esalen, in Big Sur which was established in the 1960s. Its emphasis was on therapy group settings as it related to personal growth. I visited Esalen in the mid-1980s, participating in a seminar with one of the original founders as well as a workshop focusing on gestalt therapy as it related to the mind-body connect.

Suitcase in Paradise

In a 1984 adventure, I accepted an offer to run New Life during the winter in the Caribbean. More specifically, my challenge was to inject a health-conscious dimension into the cuisine of the Prospect Reef Resort on the Island of Tortola in the British Virgin Islands. The resort had an Olympic pool, fitness classes, no massage or hiking, and daily sailing for snorkeling and excursions to the nearby islands. My assurance of my own culinary experience and adeptness in health-conscious cuisine allowed me to work productively with the kitchen staff. My self-confidence had enabled me to step into many kitchens, both before and after Tortola, to introduce kitchen practices that enhanced the healthful outcome of the menus prepared.

I equipped myself with as much health food as one of my two Tortola-bound suitcases could contain to tilt the odds of success more certainly in my favor. Soon I discovered the unhealthy food they served on the daily excursions. I boarded and inspected the boat's food supply and ordered the captain to rid the vessel of its sodas and practically all the rest of its food. Then I changed the food supply to include a large fruit salad, ak-mak crackers, cottage cheese, and tropical juices. I also had food imported from a health food store from another island.

I had created a tropical wellness paradise. As it turned out, my efforts were not unnoticed or unappreciated. Gloria Steinem, a feminist pioneer, was a guest. I had a copy of her then latest book. She signed it, "To Jimmy who is changing the world from the inside out."

Beyond the challenge of the poor food environment I faced from the Tortola experience, there is a lesson for you as well. As I did in Tortola, you are going to have to change your own kitchen environment. You must replace the food that you remove with the healthy food that will support your lifestyle transformation. I hope this story gives you another incentive to learn to select, purchase, and prepare real food that is good for your pond.

Talking the Talk

New Life and I fared well into the 1980s. Summers brought New Life between two and three hundred guests. For each coming season, I tracked the latest diet trends that guests would bring to New Life when they arrived. This enabled me to sort through and select aspects of those trends to determine the extent of adaptability to my core philosophy of serving mostly water-based foods. Even if I was in principle opposed to dieting and might not find much value in the trending diet's foods or regimens, this enabled me to address guests' interests and respond to the discussions that arose in lectures.

To meet the fitness component that, as we have seen, arose in tandem with focus on eating behavior in the 1980s, I introduced a hiking program. Stratton's variety of scenic topography permitted a different hike each day. The escalation of activity gave me the opportunity to increase meal portions for guests. As Nina and Garrett's fitness classes were becoming outdated, I made changes in the activity content and teaching techniques. I hired additional fitness staff.

New Life's purpose was to convey and apply the most qualitative knowledge possible in the pursuit of *authentic wellness*. This was to create an environment consistent with what I termed a modified Pritikin plan, calling for most of its food to come from the produce section of the grocery store. Healthy food that was delicious to eat coupled with activity provided an environment for New Life guests to become healthier and stronger. *Authentic wellness* was possible for New Life guests who could establish a daily food and fitness environment compatible with their personal lifestyles.

And Walking the Walk

At the beginning of the 1980s, I ventured out of Herbie's kitchen and into the destination spa industry. I learned about being an entrepreneur, and New Life became an established enterprise. The cook who had worked in Herbie's kitchen had become the primary source of summer revenue for the Liftline Lodge.

In the latter part of the 1980s, Herbie and Gretel were nearing retirement, and the lodge was becoming worse for its ware. Like many business, New Life was also affected by the stock market decline of the late 1980s. New Life was a big business with a large staff. Most winters I lived in New York and ran New Life in the summers. These circumstances coalesced to affirm my own sense that I had reached a new fork in the road on my journey.

It became clear to me that I needed to find a new location for New Life. My search encompassed about thirty sites from Maine to Virginia. I checked out sites recommended by many people who had been New Life guests. Often within ten minutes of looking at a recommended property, I would ask myself, "Why did they recommend this place to me? Hadn't they been to New Life? Couldn't they understand that New Life wouldn't work here?" All of this was making me feel frustrated and nervous. I wasn't finding anywhere that would present New Life as I wanted.

With the decision about a new location for New Life up in the air, I felt that I should prepare myself for a real job. I decided on a graduate school program. After considering many advanced programs, I decided against nutrition and exercise physiology. I believed that more than ten years of learning and experience with New Life's food and fitness objectives had already provided me with a good foundation in the pursuit of wellness.

I realized that my understanding of wellness required that I look more into the mental element of the mind-body connection. Food and fitness were the body aspect of this connection, and I was familiar with that. I knew that much healing was possible solely through the good foods, various forms of physical activity, and body manipulation. I began to look for a program that would focus on the mental aspect of wellness and would lead to suitable employment if the direction of my life turned that way.

With decisions about New Life's move and graduate school churning but unresolved, I moved my winter base out of New York City, where sublets had grown scarce in the late 1980s. I moved to a friend's house in Westport, Connecticut, and commuted to New York City for the marketing I did each winter. I found that I enjoyed living outside the city. It was also easier for me to look at properties.

After considering several options, I was accepted into graduate school at the University of Bridgeport. It was a three-year counseling program. At the conclusion I could become an employment assistance program (EAP) counselor. Counselor positions with corporations had opened as EAPs were established to assist employees with a wide range of personal issues.

New Life in the summer now cycled over to off-season life in Connecticut, where I lived and attended graduate school. I loved and so benefited from the graduate school courses. To my own great satisfaction, my graduate studies in counseling at the University of Bridgeport allowed me to place the therapeutic process under a figurative electronic microscope. I became immersed in a wide range of therapeutic modalities. This understanding gave me the opportunity to learn how to work in a therapeutic setting, helping clients with the pattern and behaviors that had created unhealthy lifestyle situations.

While I was a graduate student, the renowned psychologist Dr. Albert Ellis, who developed rational emotive behavior therapy, came to our school for a guest lecture. During Dr. Ellis's presentation, I was invited on stage to participate in a demonstration of his therapeutic techniques. Very quickly, my discussion and his commentary focused on the emotion I was expressing about the nature of my childhood relationship with my mother. To my surprise, Dr. Ellis interrupted me almost immediately and asked me if my mother was still alive. I said no. Dr. Ellis questioned quickly, "And the problem is?"

Our interaction ended abruptly at that moment. No further discussion or elaboration was necessary. Moreover, neither I nor anyone else could escape the point that his technique had made. My problem could no longer have anything to do with my late mother, who had died many years earlier. My thoughts were irrational. My problem had only to do with me. Fossilized in my emotional structure were remnants of childhood pain that had nothing to do with my present life situation.

The clarity and power of these succinct moments with Dr. Ellis had both immediate and future therapeutic benefits. For me, the pain would remain always fresh unless I engaged my adult awareness in dissolving and letting go of the lingering emotional filters that were self-prohibitive and self-limiting.

Consequently, after completion of my MS degree in counseling in 1992 at the University of Bridgeport, I established a nutritional coaching practice in New York City. Structurally, my nutritional coaching program would be a short-term, ten-session therapeutic approach toward healthy eating. It was designed to communicate an overview of a low-fat, high-complex carbohydrate basis for healthy eating. Conceptually, I would examine eating, the most essential and primary human behavior, in terms of education, psychology, and sociology of eating. Through behavioral, cognitive, and insight therapy, the individual would acquire an understanding of the mind-body framework required for changes in eating habits. Within this understanding, the individual would begin to evaluate and restructure their relationship with their food environment, including refrigerators, cupboards, food shopping locations, and their family, social, and business lives.

The following is the letter I sent to my mailing list of New Life guests in Manhattan in 1993, explaining nutritional coaching. I was ahead of my time.

Since college, I have always dealt with life situations in a dimensional way. My development of New Life and nutritional coaching illustrated that. Nutritional coaching gives the framework that will transform eating and fitness patterns to create *authentic wellness*. That is the foundation of this book.

My over 20 years of experience and training as an expert chef, founder and director of New Life Hiking Spa®, and MS in Counseling has led me to offer you a common-sense realistic approach toward healthy eating that I call "Nutritional Coaching".

Nutritional Coaching is based on a short term (10 to 12 sessions) therapeutic approach that will include:

1. An over view of what food is and the relationship between the different fats, complex and simple carbohydrates, and protein. **The Education of Eating.**
2. Using behavioral-cognitive and insight therapy, you gain the insight and perspective to build the body/mind framework for changes in eating habits. **The Psychology of Eating.**
3. Evaluate and restructure your relationship with your food environment. This included: your refrigerator and cupboards, your grocery and health food store and your social and business life. **The Sociology of Eating.**

As I worked with the individuals I coached, I was very impressed with the gains they achieved. Of course, I received the benefits from the therapeutic relationship as well. I learned that most people have a basic understanding of foods that are and are not healthy. Within therapy, however, unlike the familiar all-or-nothing diet regimen for weight loss, I did not suggest that a person had to give up his or her favorite food, and weight loss was not an objective or concern either. Instead the individual made changes from examining his or her lifestyle.

Together, the nutritional coaching and New Life experiences helped me understand the dimensions of the process of changing eating habits. I found that changing eating habits was not a linear process but a subjective and multifaceted one. I learned that the individual's ability to make the changes was enhanced by identifying his or her subjective reason(s) for resisting the change, the person's psychology of eating. Once they began to understand the sources of their resistance to change, they could work on reprogramming how they perceived their eating habits to make the lifestyle changes they desired.

Crossing the Divide

As I was absorbed in my graduate studies, I learned about a new possibility for New Life at Killington, Vermont. I had already been to Killington and didn't know of anything suitable there. I realized that I had become partial to Vermont because of its natural beauty and the personal growth and successes I had experienced there. I understood my genuine attachment to Vermont when, during one winter in my Manhattan apartment, I awoke from a dream where I was gazing into the unmatched summer green of Vermont's hills and valleys. Finally, Vermont's beckoning for me to stay came as a recommendation from a source in whom, ironically, I had little regard for but one who convinced me to look at an inn in Killington, Vermont. Turned out it was the right fit for New Life, and I moved New Life to Killington in 1992. I decided to continue to be an entrepreneur rather than a therapist. I feel very positive about my decision and have kept New Life going throughout the 1990s into the twenty-first-century. After all these years, I have been encouraged that the food philosophy I developed forty year ago has passed the test of time.

What More?

I have become a wellness expert. As a wellness expert, I cannot overspecialize. There are so many dimensions to wellness, and the interaction among them is exceedingly subtle, personal, and subjective. Like the water from which all life comes, wellness is a flow. The substance of wellness is real food, the essence of which is water-based. To attain authentic wellness, we must address our relationship with food in an innovate fashion that bears in mind the complex and personalized lifestyles of the twenty-first century.

Through New Life, I will continue to offer participants the opportunity for a healthy respite in the central mountains of Vermont. I will offer those New Life participants already engaged in lifestyle transformation an opportunity to reignite their motivation. I will offer New Life participants not yet engaged in their own lifestyle transformations the inspiration and guidance to start. I offer this life narrative to convey the experiences that formed my beliefs on the pursuit of wellness.

What more is there for me to do? The message offered about *authentic wellness* has been delivered personally by me to the New Life participant. Consistent with the advice once given to me by the Zuckerman's of Canyon Ranch, I remain the energy source of New Life. My ability to remain as that source is possible largely due to the personal and professional quality of service rendered by the New Life staff.

Along with running New Life, I believe that I can do more to convey the New Life message across a broader panorama than has yet been the case. Businesses and organizations of all varieties and sizes have become attentive to the wellness of their employees and members.

Accordingly, I believe that there is a niche that New Life can fill in applying the concepts of its food philosophy to the existing business and organizational wellness programs. New Life food philosophy is also applicable to the in-house food preparation and meals served by businesses, schools, hospitals, and other organizations. I have collaborated, critiqued, and worked with kitchen and food preparation managers and staff to reform operations that, without additional cost consequences, will support employee efforts to understand and transform food related behavior to create *Authentic Wellness*.

ABOUT THE AUTHOR

James T. LeSage, always known as "Jimmy", is the founder and, for 40 years, owner and operator, of the New Life Hiking Spa® in the Green Mountains of central Vermont. At New Life, no one else ever answers the telephone for reservations or inquiries.

Jimmy's life as a nutrition and fitness professional yields practical wisdom individually transferrable to the reader's lifestyle. Without diets or directives, he calls us to an Authentic Wellness by reconceiving our multi-dimensional and complex relationship with food.

Jimmy received a B.A. from Florida State University and M.S. in Counseling from the University of Bridgeport.